PROVIDING
COMMUNITY-BASED
SERVICES TO THE
RURAL ELDERLY

OTHER RECENT VOLUMES IN THE
SAGE FOCUS EDITIONS

PROVIDING COMMUNITY-BASED SERVICES TO THE RURAL ELDERLY

John A. Krout
editor

SAGE PUBLICATIONS
International Educational and Professional Publisher
Thousand Oaks   London   New Delhi

For information address:

SAGE Publications, Inc.
2455 Teller Road
Thousand Oaks, California 91320

SAGE Publications Ltd.
6 Bonhill Street
London EC2A 4PU
United Kingdom

SAGE Publications India Pvt. Ltd.
M-32 Market
Greater Kailash I
New Delhi 110 048 India

Printed in the United States of America

Library of Congress Cataloging-in-Publication Data

Main entry under title:

Providing community-based services to the rural elderly / John A.
    Krout, editor.
        p.   cm. — (Sage focus edition ; 165)
    Includes bibliographical references and indexes.
    ISBN 0–8039–4695–3. — ISBN 0–8039–4696–1 (pbk.)
        1. Rural aged—Services for—United States. 2. Rural aged—United
States.   I. Krout, John A.   II. Series: Sage focus editions ; vol.
165.
    HV1461.P79   1993
    362.6′3′0973—dc20   93–31226
                                                                                       CIP

94   95   96   97   10   9   8   7   6   5   4   3   2   1

Sage Production Editor: Yvonne Könneker

Contents

To the thousands of practitioners and volunteers working to better the lives of older rural persons through the provision of community-based services.

Preface

This book attempts to bring together information from both researchers and practitioners on community-based services for the rural elderly. The purpose is to present detailed and specific information on a wide range of community-based services that are needed by and available to varying degrees to elders living in rural areas. The focus is on exploring how these services can be developed and provided given the realities of rural settings, resources, and populations. Where appropriate, rural/urban comparisons are made, but the focus is on the status of rural older populations and the ways in which their needs are and can best be met by a variety of community-based programs. Although it is generally acknowledged that rural areas support fewer services for older persons and that rural service access problems are considerable, many rural programs do meet the needs of the elderly. This volume draws on the expertise of researchers and practitioners—two groups that often do not communicate and thus do not understand or appreciate what each can learn from the other.

This book has several major goals. The first is to present research-based information on rural elderly community service provision that is useful to and usable by practitioners, planners, and policy makers. Thus, although the contributors do identify barriers to the development and operation of community-based services for older rural persons, the focus is on programmatic responses and solutions to service needs and barriers. Another goal is to identify both practice and policy gaps and needs. A third goal is to further interdisciplinary and research/practice "cross-fertilization" of ideas and expertise. A fourth goal is to identify applied research needs and policy issues in rural gerontology. Finally, it should be stressed that this is not a "how to" book or a manual on service provision, although it includes many useful insights on program development and operation. Rather, it is a presentation of program ideas and observations that can assist rural service practitioners. The bottom line is to further the understanding of how a range of community-based services can best be provided to the rural elderly.

Coverage in This Volume

A broad range of topics is covered here, including most of the areas considered to be formal "community-based" services. Obviously, informal networks provide large amounts—indeed, the majority—of community-based care for the rural elderly. However, there is already a considerable body of research on the activities of informal support networks and caregivers—although not enough focused on rural areas—and the breadth of topics included under the "formal" heading, combined with length limitations, precluded a focus on rural informal networks. They are referred to where appropriate.

Part I of the book presents an introductory chapter that reviews the general status and needs of older rural populations and the availability of community-based services for the rural elderly. The specific formal community-based services covered in this book are grouped into three sections. Part II covers information and referral, transportation, case management, and senior centers. Part III examines housing, employment and retirement, and respite and adult day care. Part IV explores nutrition, health and wellness promotion, in-home health care, and mental health. The book closes with an epilogue that provides an overview of common themes and issues in rural community-based service provision.

Of course, other topics could have been included, but I had to choose between covering a larger number of topics superficially and including a smaller number in greater depth to stay within the publisher's length guidelines. Where information is available, the chapters refer to the unique circumstances and needs of populations most likely to be at risk, such as minority and low-income elderly.

The Approach Taken

The coverage of topics makes this volume comprehensive in terms of community-based services. As noted above, both research and application are covered, but the major thrust is service development and provision. It is assumed that the needs are there and that existing responses to these needs are, overall, inadequate, as is the existing knowledge base for practitioners and researchers alike. Chapters include a combination of reviews of the research literature and information on programming. However, the book is not a collection of examples, with individuals relating only their own experiences.

All the chapters follow the same basic format and organization of material. Although individual authors approached their topics differently, the chapters all include the following elements: a brief review of the scope, nature, and need for a specific service (the need the service addresses); standard and alternative approaches to meeting the need; problems encountered in developing and providing the service; core elements of successful approaches; an overview of research and policy issues; and a summary and conclusions section. Most chapters are co-authored, with one author coming from primarily a research background and one coming from a practitioner perspective. In some cases, individuals have been found who combine both of these. The research perspective is "applied," not basic, so theoretical questions—say, about inter-/intraorganizational dynamics or costs of services—are not covered.

As far as I know, no book currently exists with the same focus as this one. There are many books on community-based services for the elderly in general, but none that concentrates on the *rural* elderly. There are several books on the rural elderly that focus on the status and characteristics of this population and that are written primarily from a research perspective (see, e.g., Bull, 1993; Coward & Lee, 1985a; Coward, Bull, Kukulka, & Galliher, in press; Kim & Wilson, 1981; Krout, 1986). Although important and of value, none of these works attempts to combine research and practice while focusing on service provision. Thus this book is distinguished by both its topic (service planning and provision to the rural elderly) and its approach (comprehensive and applied, with a basis in existing research).

The primary intended audience for this volume is made up of practitioners, planners, and policy makers who are working, or preparing to work, in the area of rural aging and community-based health and social services for the elderly. The book should also be useful to policy planners and administrators in general, who often have little background in rural aging issues. Other possible audiences include rural and gerontological researchers with "applied" interests as well as educators teaching courses in gerontology, rural health, and a wide range of disciplines (social work, allied health professions). It is my hope that graduate and undergraduate course instructors and students in aging services development, planning, and provision will find this book of interest. Ideally, this work will be found useful in technical assistance and continuing education instruction for rural practitioners.

—John A. Krout

Acknowledgments

I would first and foremost like to acknowledge the contributors to this volume for their hard work, perseverance, and expertise. They have given unselfishly of their time and energy to make this book a reality. Second, as always, my spouse deserves recognition for her unflagging support and tolerance of an often cranky editor. The demands of book writing inevitably place strains on one's home life, but Bobbi Krout has born these with more patience and good cheer than imaginable. Finally, I would like to thank Sage Publications, and in particular Christine Smedley, for having confidence in my ideas for this book, and for providing expert assistance in all aspects of the development and production of this work.

PART I

Overview of the Rural Elderly

This section, which contains a single chapter, presents an overview of the rural elderly. The chapter begins with a brief discussion of some of the ambiguity that surrounds the definition of the term *rural* in the literature, and argues that the diversity that makes up rural settings must be recognized, and that a continuum of residence based on a number of factors is perhaps the best approach. Data on the sociodemographic makeup of older rural populations are also provided.

Chapter 1 offers discussion of a number of myths about the rural elderly that revolve around the fact that many people believe rural elders to be better off than elders living in cities. It is demonstrated that these idealized rural images do not fit with reality. Older rural populations have lower incomes and are more likely to live in poverty, to live in older and more substandard housing, and to face greater transportation difficulties than their urban counterparts. There is also evidence that the rural elderly experience poorer health in a number of areas.

These difficulties provide the basis for the rural elderly's need for community-based services. However, a number of obstacles have combined to reduce the extent to which these services have been able to meet the elderly's needs. Lack of resources, access difficulties brought about by low population densities and a lack of transportation, low levels of service awareness, and a resistance to admitting need and accepting services among the rural elderly are just some of the obstacles identified in Chapter 1. Rural community-based service providers must overcome challenges related to service availability, accessibility, awareness, acceptability, affordability, appropriateness, and adequacy.

The chapter ends with an overview of what, in general, is known about community-based services for the rural elderly. Rural older

1

persons have access to a smaller number and narrower range of these services, even though the rural-urban gap in this regard may have diminished somewhat in recent years. Significant gaps exist in the "continuum of care" in many rural communities, although considerable variation is found in service availability and accessibility among rural communities. Very little attention has been paid to careful analysis of the causes of these residence differences and to the development and evaluation of rural service delivery models and strategies. Few service professionals have been trained to respond to the unique circumstances and dynamics of rural communities, and much more attention needs to be focused on enhancing the skills of rural practitioners. It also appears that some regulatory and reimbursement policies impede the development and provision of rural community-based services. The chapter concludes with an argument that the need for more detailed information on this topic and on how community-based services can best be supported and provided to rural elders provides the basic rationale for this book.

1

An Overview of
Older Rural Populations
and Community-Based Services

JOHN A. KROUT

What Is Rural?

Before we begin our investigation of individual community-based services, it is important to clarify our use of the word *rural*. A discussion
of what is meant by this term and of the characteristics of older persons
living in rural places will set the stage for subsequent chapters. Research
on rural aging has incorporated many different definitions of *rural* (see
Krout & Dwyer, 1991, for an expanded discussion). Traditionally, and
unfortunately, many considerations of rural aging issues have adopted
rural/urban or nonmetropolitan/metropolitan dichotomies based on population size (U.S. Department of Agriculture, 1984). According to such
classifications, rural communities are considered to be those having populations of fewer than 2,500 people. But population size is not the only
salient variable in defining whether an area is rural. Population density,
as in the "frontier" designation of areas with fewer than six persons per
square mile (Popper, 1986), and typologies that include metropolitan
status as well as proximity to metropolitan areas have also been used
(Hines, Brown, & Zimmer, 1975). In addition, occupational structure
also differentiates communities. Most familiar to rural observers is the
farm/nonfarm distinction (U.S. Department of Agriculture, 1985).

These definitions help illustrate the considerable diversity that exists within what is generally called "rural America." Moreover, this definitional smorgasbord is complicated by the fact that these various definitions are not generally or necessarily mutually exclusive. For example, 30% of the *rural* population in this country resides within *metropolitan* counties (Hassinger, 1982). Clearly, the conceptualization of residence as a dichotomous variable does not fit with the reality and diversity of residential settings that range from central cities to open rangeland. Place of residence is best conceptualized as a continuum, from most rural to most urban. Rural America encompasses a rich diversity that stretches from the woods of Maine to the Mississippi delta and from the hollows of Appalachia to the desert and rangeland of the great Southwest.

For this examination of community-based services, residence should be viewed as a continuum including number and density of population, distance from population centers, and a core set of services and an economic structure that are likely to be tied, historically and currently, to extractive industries, such as farming, mining, and lumbering. In spite of the issues noted above, the contributors to this book use the term *rural* generically to refer to a continuum of residential environments outside of cities and suburbs. Where the data are available and appropriate, metropolitan versus nonmetropolitan, rural versus urban, and farm versus nonfarm categories are used.

How Many Rural Elderly?

The number of elderly in the United States counted as rural depends on the particular definition of *rural* one uses. Data from the 1990 census reveal that 8.2 million older persons live in nonmetropolitan areas (26% of the total elderly population) and 23 million live in metropolitan places (U.S. Senate, Special Committee on Aging, 1992). Some 90% of the rural elderly are reported to *not* be living on farms, underscoring the fact that the term *rural* is no longer indicative of residence on a farm. As of 1988, it was estimated that about 700,000, or only 2.5% of the total elderly population, lived on farms. However, it is likely that this figure undercounts the true number, because the definition of *farm residence* used by the U.S. Census Bureau includes only households with at least $1,000 in income from the sale of agricultural products. Thus elders living on farms that do not meet this criterion would not be counted as farm residents (Coward & Dwyer, 1991a; Krout & Dwyer, 1991).

Generally speaking, the proportion of the population age 65 and over increases as the overall population of a place decreases. In 1980, the highest proportion of elderly (15.4%) was found for small towns in rural areas, and the lowest proportion (10.0%) was found for urban fringe or suburban areas of urbanized territory. By 1990, the elderly made up 15% of the nonmetropolitan but only 12% of the metropolitan population (U.S. Senate, Special Committee on Aging, 1992). The higher percentage of elderly found in small towns has been attributed to several factors, such as the out-migration of young adults, the "aging in place" of middle-aged cohorts, and the movement of retired farmers and especially widows of farmers to somewhat larger communities (Siegel, 1979). This out-migration traditionally has been viewed in terms of its negative consequences for rural economies, but it also may leave those elderly "left behind" with fewer social contacts and more limited support systems (Deimling & Huber, 1981). Rural communities, with their higher elderly dependency ratios, also face the additional task of supporting programs and services for these elders.

Important differences exist also at the regional level in the numbers and proportions of rural elderly. As of 1980, 43.0% of the nation's nonmetropolitan elderly lived in the South and 32.6% lived in the North Central states; only 13.2% resided in the Northeast and 10.8% in the West (Krout, 1986). This pattern of regional differences has likely not changed in the early 1990s. Variation is also found at the state level; some states are much more likely than others to have significant rural elderly populations. For example, as of 1980 the states with the highest concentrations of elderly in totally rural counties were Kansas, Iowa, Missouri, and Nebraska (all 18% or more). The states with the lowest proportions of elderly in rural counties were Alaska, Colorado, Louisiana, Maryland, Nevada, and New Mexico (4.1%-9.6%) (Clifford, Heaton, Voss, & Fuguitt, 1985). In many states, significant percentages of the elderly live in rural areas, making rural issues an important part of aging policy and programs. As of 1980, a majority of the elderly in 21 states and two-fifths of the elderly in 28 states lived in rural areas (Harbert & Wilkinson, 1979; Kim, 1981).

Characteristics of the Rural Elderly

It is a well-accepted tenet in gerontology that sociodemographic characteristics are important factors that must be considered in policy decisions, program development, and service provision. Certain sociodemographic characteristics are strongly correlated with and often used as proxies for particular health and social needs. For example, the proportion of elderly reporting difficulty performing activities of daily living has generally been found to increase with age and to be greater for females, nonwhites, and persons with lower incomes (Kart, 1991). Thus it is important not only to know how many elderly live in rural areas of the United States but also to have knowledge of their sociodemographic characteristics, such as age, race, sex, marital status, and household composition. Each of these factors has generally been found to covary with residence and thus affects the need for community-based services.

Age

We have seen that the proportion of the total population that is elderly is greater in smaller places than in larger places. However, that does not necessarily mean that a similar rural/urban difference exists for the age distribution among the elderly. Indeed, Coward, McLaughlin, Duncan, and Bull (1992) report data from the 1991 Current Population Survey (CPS) that show nonmetropolitan areas have higher percentages of population in the 65-74 age group than do non-central-city metropolitan and total metropolitan areas, and higher percentages in the 75-84 age group than do non-central-city metropolitan areas. No residence differences were found in the proportion of population 85 years and older. Thus, although there are rural communities that have relatively high proportions of elderly in the older age groups, this is not the case nationally. In addition, Coward, McLaughlin, et al. (1992) found that nonmetropolitan areas have a higher "dependency ratio" (the number of persons under age 18 and over age 64, divided by the number in the 19-64 age range) than any other residence category. Thus working-age persons face a potentially greater burden for services for the elderly in nonmetropolitan areas.

Race

In terms of race, data for the elderly by residence are limited and can be criticized because of inconsistencies in how racial groups are categorized. For example, sometimes Hispanics are grouped with "whites" and sometimes with "nonwhites." Data on distinct Hispanic groups (e.g., Mexican American, Cuban American, Puerto Rican) are rarely provided for the elderly overall, and residence breakdowns are not available at this level of detail. Clearly, however, the distribution of different racial and ethnic groups by residence varies dramatically. Overall, in 1990 about 656,000 nonwhite elders lived in nonmetropolitan areas versus almost 2.7 million in metropolitan areas (U.S. Senate, Special Committee on Aging, 1992). As of 1990, more than one-half million nonmetropolitan elders were classified as African Americans; 132,000 were classified as Hispanics (of any race); 61,000 were American Indians, Eskimos, or Aleuts; 33,000 were Asian and Pacific Islanders; and 38,000 were of other races (U.S. Senate, Special Committee on Aging, 1992). Nonmetropolitan areas generally have higher percentages of whites and lower percentages of blacks than do metropolitan areas (especially central cities). Further, nonmetropolitan areas have more black but fewer Hispanic elders than do non-central-city areas (Coward, McLaughlin, et al., 1992). It also should be pointed out that the vast majority (93.5%) of black nonmetropolitan elderly live in the South (Parks, 1988).

In 1990, the majority of Asian and Pacific Islanders and Hispanics lived in metropolitan areas, but the majority of American Indians, Eskimos, and Aleuts lived in nonmetropolitan areas (U.S. Senate, Special Committee on Aging, 1992). Depending on the region of the country, rural areas have different concentrations of racial minorities. For example, Hispanics are prominent in the rural Southwest. However, published data on rural Hispanics or Native Americans older persons are very difficult to find.

Sex and Marital Status

As for the sex structure of the elderly population, it is well known that there are more females than males among this group. This is generally illustrated by the use of the "sex ratio"—the number of male elderly per 100 female elderly. The 1991 CPS data reveal higher sex ratios for rural areas: 69.6 for metropolitan versus 76.9 for nonmetropolitan, with metropolitan central cities reporting the lowest figure (64.1) (Coward, McLaughlin, et al., 1992). These sex ratio differences by residence may be attributed in part to sex-specific migration patterns of widowed rural elderly females (especially in sparsely populated areas), who often move to larger communities when their health status and ability to live independently decline. We would expect them to be mirrored by residential differences in marital status and living arrangements of the elderly.

Such patterns are displayed in the 1991 CPS data. Coward, McLaughlin, et al. (1992) report that nonmetropolitan older persons in every age category are more likely to be married (and less likely to be widowed, divorced, or separated) than are central-city elders. Living arrangements show corresponding residence differences. Nonmetropolitan elderly in every age category are also more likely to be living in husband-wife households than are central-city elders and are less likely to live in female-headed households (Coward, McLaughlin, et al., 1992).

These data suggest a rural advantage in the availability of informal family support (especially a spouse), a major factor in avoiding or delaying the institutionalization of frail elders as well as the overall quality of life of the elderly (Coward, McLaughlin, et al., 1992). But they should not be interpreted as indicating that there is no need for formal community-based services. As is the case for metropolitan elders, marriage rates and presence of a spouse for nonmetropolitan elders decline dramatically in the older age groups (85 and older). Indeed, one could argue that nonmetropolitan elderly households may be more likely to have spouses involved in caregiving who have needs for assistance from community-based services that may not be available. This rural community-based service disadvantage, not just the greater likelihood of marriage, may account for the finding reported by Coward, Cutler, and Mullens (1990) that nonmetropolitan as opposed to metropolitan disabled elders are more likely to receive informal assistance only.

Myths of Rural Aging

Integral to our understanding of who the rural elderly are and of their need for community-based services is a brief examination of the misconceptions and myths that surround this population. In general, rural elders are often seen as whiling away their final years in bucolic farm settings, living in large houses surrounded by an abundance of fresh air, food, supportive neighbors, and a large, loving extended family ready to provide help when the need arises. Let us look at the various components of this myth. First, although not rich, rural elders are better able than others to "make ends meet" because a lifetime "down on the farm" has taught them to provide for many of their own basic needs (such as gardening and making clothes). Second, rural elders are healthier, having been toughened by a lifetime of physical labor and blessed by their less hectic, less stressful lifestyle. Third, rural elders are generally happier than their urban counterparts because of their "wealth" and health, and because they are satisfied with the "basics" in life (i.e., they desire fewer materials things than do elders living in urban areas). Fourth, rural elders do not need or want the same formal services as do other older populations because they are healthier and happier, and because they have those large extended families living nearby to provide them with assistance should it ever become necessary. Rural communities are also seen as well integrated, with a common value structure that provides support and assistance to older persons in need. Finally, older rural populations are seen as homogeneous in terms of sociodemographic characteristics.

The reality, as the chapters that follow illustrate, is far from this romantic, idealized stereotype. Although many rural elders have lived in or near farming communities for significant parts of their lives, very few currently live on farms. Housing problems and deficiencies abound for rural elders, and that old farmhouse, where it does exist, is expensive to maintain and generally a totally inappropriate living environment for elders as they become more frail with increasing age. Rural elders face income deficits and are much more likely to be poor than are elders living elsewhere. Overall, nonfarm rural elders appear to be less healthy than metropolitan residents and to live in environments with far fewer health care facilities and professionals per capita than do other elders. Rural elders in need of health and social services face problems in service availability and accessibility, and those with severe impairments often must travel long distances to receive medical specialty care. They must rely on private vehicles because of limited public transportation alternatives.

Many rural elderly do not use services, but this is not because of a lack of need, but because the services are either nonexistent or limited in scope and affordability. Informal helping networks for the elderly are not necessarily larger in rural areas, and geographic distance from—not proximity to—nonspousal informal helpers further mitigates the supposed rural advantage. Rural elders are not more satisfied with their life circumstances than are other older persons, they apparently just do not report being less satisfied. Generic or "one size fits all" programmatic responses are not appropriate for rural elders, and programs that work in one rural area may have little attractiveness or impact in other rural places.

Problems Facing the Rural Elderly

Income and Poverty

Numerous studies have shown that rural elders have lower incomes than their urban counterparts (Coward & Lee, 1985a; Krout, 1986). Indeed, they are reported to be approximately 20% lower than those of the metropolitan elderly, reflecting lower social security payments, smaller savings, less widespread coverage by private pensions, fewer opportunities for part-time work, and infrequent enrollment in SSI (Krout, 1986). It is also important to point out that the elderly make up a greater percentage of the poor in rural areas (Porter, 1989).

As would be expected given these data, rural elders are more likely to be poor than are nonrural elders. As of 1987, half of the nonmetropolitan versus 37% of the metropolitan elderly lived in families that had incomes below or within 200% of the poverty line (U.S. Senate, Special Committee on Aging, 1992). Data from 1989 reveal that the nonmetropolitan poverty rate for those 65 years old and older was 15% versus 10% for the metropolitan elderly (U.S. Bureau of the Census, 1991a), with 34% of nonmetropolitan black males, 46% of nonmetropolitan black females, and 34% of nonmetropolitan white females living under the poverty line. Another way to see the extent of poverty among the rural elderly is to focus on households. In 1985, 27% of nonmetropolitan households headed by persons 65 and older were poor, with two-thirds of poor nonmetropolitan households consisting of individuals living alone (mostly women) (Lazere et al., 1989).

However, 1991 Current Population Survey data demonstrate that there are no significant poverty rate differences between central-city and nonmetropolitan elderly, but that the nonmetropolitan rates for both these residence categories are higher than those for non-central-city elders (Coward, McLaughlin, et al., 1992). The rural elderly income disadvantage is not surprising, given that rural poverty rates have historically been higher than urban rates (Fitchen, 1990). Although the majority of the nonmetropolitan elderly poor have been poor for most of their lives, some have become poor during their older years as a result of declining income or major health problems (Coward, McLaughlin, et al., 1992).

The nonmetropolitan elderly income and poverty disadvantage has significant implications for the ability of this population to meet health and social needs and the need for services. Poorer people generally have experienced poorer health and less access to adequate health care throughout their lives. Thus older rural residents would appear to have substantial needs in the areas of income support and health services.

Housing

The large majority of those living in nonmetropolitan elderly households (80%) are homeowners, with most of their houses having been built before 1940. These elders have lived in their homes longer than have metropolitan residents (Krout, 1986), and their houses are more likely to lack modern heating systems and plumbing facilities, to be uninsulated, and to be in need of costly repairs. Data from the 1970s and 1980s indicate that the overall quality of rural elderly housing is worse than urban housing as measured by lack or insufficiency of basic necessities and presence of undesirable features (Bylund, LeRay, & Crawford, 1980; Krout, 1986). Thus the quality of their housing presents impaired elders with a higher level of "environmental press" (Lawton & Nahemow, 1973), which may necessitate relocation to a more accommodating environment. The need for home repair programs as well as attention to increasing the housing options available to older persons is manifest.

Transportation

Available and affordable access to services and the amenities of life has been shown to be one of the most important concerns of rural elders as well as one of the most difficult problems for service providers to overcome (Krout, 1986, 1989a). The basic problem is a lack of alternatives to the privately owned vehicle, especially a paucity of public transportation systems in rural areas. Rural elders have much higher rates of vehicle ownership than do their urban counterparts (Cutler & Coward, 1992) and thus are more likely to bear the costs associated with running and maintaining such vehicles. But the mere presence of a vehicle does not eliminate transportation problems, especially for those frail elders who have difficulty negotiating the long distances between services and people characteristic of rural areas.

Access problems also add time and expense to service delivery efforts and discourage the development of new services and expansion of existing services into rural areas. Some rural directors of Area Agencies on Aging (AAAs), for example, have observed that the expense of running basic transportation systems for congregate and in-home programs significantly limits the amount of resources available for the services themselves (Krout, 1989a). City-based in-home service providers, for example, may not be able to justify (in terms of profit) providing services in low-density rural areas with large distances between relatively few clients. The lack of transportation increases the difficulty and cost of accessing special medical care increasingly available only in larger population centers. In sum, access difficulties underlie virtually all of the circumstances of older rural populations and present a considerable challenge to community-based service providers.

Health

Many studies indicate a rural health status disadvantage as well as less availability and accessibility of health care professionals and services. It has been documented consistently that rural areas have fewer health resources and a lower ratio of doctors, nurses, pharmacists, and so on to population than do urban areas (Coward, McLaughlin, et al., 1992; Krout, 1986). Rural hospitals continue to have higher closure rates and to be at greater risk of closure than urban hospitals experiencing low occupancy rates and high uncollected charges (Riley & Elder, 1991).

In general, the research suggests that rural and urban older persons have similar health problems, but rural elders have higher rates of chronic disease, including arthritis, cardiovascular diseases, hypertension, and diabetes (Krout, 1986). As is the case with other health indicators, the data rarely show a linear relationship between health status and population size or community type, nor are differences universal across all health measures (Coward, McLaughlin, et al., 1992). For example, Coward, Miller, and Dwyer (1992) analyzed data for 26 health measures from the 1984-1986 Longitudinal Supplement of Aging of the National Health Interview and found significant residential differences for 16 of the measures. Three-quarters of these showed a rural disadvantage, including the total number of functional limitations, more limitations with particular functions (e.g., walking, reaching over the head), and a greater percentage noting the presence of some medical conditions (e.g., hypertension, arthritis, accidental falls). Rural elders were also more likely to indicate that their health was poor.

Several analyses of health differences by residence have found significant variation within rural categories, especially in the area of farm/nonfarm comparisons (Coward & Cutler, 1988; Coward,

McLaughlin, et al., 1992; Coward, Miller, & Dwyer, 1992). Farm elders are consistently found to report fewer activity limitations and medical conditions than do nonfarm dwellers, although they also are more likely to view their health as poor than are urban elders. Indeed, nonfarm rural elderly would appear to have the poorest health status of any residential grouping. So, nonfarm rural elders have the greatest and farm elders the smallest number of chronic conditions, but farm elders experience more acute health conditions than do other residence groups. Farm elders also report fewer days of restricted activity and fewer days in bed than do rural nonfarm elders. Yet, rural elders, especially those living on farms, see their health as worse compared with that of other older persons. Several studies of activities of daily living (ADLs) and instrumental activities of daily living (IADLs) have not found consistent rural-urban distribution for specific tasks. Farm dwellers have been found to have the smallest number of these with restrictions and rural nonfarm elders the highest, with metropolitan elders in between.

The importance of residence in determining health status independent of demographic characteristics (or compositional effects) such as income, gender, and marital status is not completely understood, but several studies have found that residence drops out as a predictor of some reported health problems when certain demographic characteristics are included (Coward & Cutler, 1988). Nonetheless, the important point for our purposes is that regardless of the cause, rural elderly health status, especially among those in the nonfarm category (which makes up the greatest proportion of rural residents by far), appears to be lower than that found among the urban elderly. This means that rural elders have a greater need for the community-based services discussed in this book, most of which are less likely to be available and accessible in rural areas.

Rural Elders and Community-Based Services

Community-based services include a broad range of services provided outside of institutional settings that help maintain the independent health and functioning of older people in a variety of ways. Services traditionally defined as community based include home care (home health, personal care, homemaker), nutrition services (congregate and in-home), mental health, information and referral/outreach, case management, senior centers, respite care, adult day care, housing, and transportation. These services complement institutional medical and long-term care services to form a continuum or array of services that ranges from family caregiving to nursing homes and, in theory, meets the needs of older people with a range of health and social needs.

Community-based services are not appropriate or cost-efficient for all needs (e.g., intensive medical treatment requiring specialized equipment and physician care), but generally are seen as less costly than hospital or nursing home care and allow individuals to remain at home, by far the preferred environment among seniors, to receive care. They also are often the only option for older persons who lack available or appropriate informal care networks and who are not impaired enough to need institutional care.

Need for Community-Based Services

As noted above, much of the literature on the status and needs of older rural persons indicates that community-based services are both needed and appropriate for them. For example, research suggests that rural older persons are more likely to have difficulties with ADLs and IADLs than are their urban counterparts (Coward & Cutler, 1988; Cutler & Coward, 1988; Krout, 1989b). Because most rural older persons experience chronic health problems that do not require long hospital stays or admission to nursing homes, community-based services can assist them in functioning as independently as possible in their own home. Community-based services also can complement the support provided by informal networks and provide care when such networks are either not available or unable/unwilling to engage in primary caregiving. It is important to note that research has shown that rural older persons, contrary to existing stereotypes, do not have larger family support networks or more contact with their adult children than do urban elderly (Krout, 1986, 1988c; Lassey & Lassey, 1985). Thus the need for community-based services in rural areas is no less than it is in urban places; indeed, as we shall see, it is arguably greater, given the more disadvantaged status of rural older persons.

Obstacles to Rural Community-Based Services

Rural older persons face problems in accessing services located in their own as well as more distant communities because of lower incomes and especially lack of transportation and transportation alternatives. Research suggests that the rural elderly have lower levels of service awareness as well and are somewhat mistrustful of and uncomfortable with the service bureaucracy, especially when it is staffed by people who do not understand rural culture and attitudes or know how to present and provide services that are culturally appropriate (Coward, 1979; Krout, 1988a; Rowles, 1991). Because community-based services are generally rooted in community social support systems and are usually provided in or near the client's community, they have the potential to overcome such problems and effectively meet the needs of diverse rural populations. For example, many small rural communities have their own senior centers staffed by local professionals and volunteers. Other service providers often employ "locals" who understand the value and normative systems of older persons and their families and are able to determine how existing services can best be presented and provided to them.

As I and others have observed, often rural communities and service systems face a lack of resources (including money and service infrastructure) and specialty staff (trained labor pool) that impedes the development of comprehensive and coordinated community-based services and leads to gaps in the so-called continuum of care (see, e.g., Fortinsky, 1991; Krout, 1986, 1992). The geographic isolation of the elderly that characterizes many rural communities, the inability to use economies of scale, and a lack of effective advocacy coalitions have also slowed the development of rural community-based services.

Overall, rural community-based services must overcome challenges posed by availability, accessibility, awareness, acceptability, affordability, appropriateness, and adequacy (Krout, 1986; Williams, Ebrite, & Redford, 1991). Indeed, the chapters that follow detail problems in these areas for virtually every service that is examined. It is generally believed that many services are not as likely to be found in rural areas (*availability*) and that the larger distances between the services that do exist and the people who need them result in higher provision costs in terms of time and money (*accessibility*). Services that are available may be incomplete or of poor quality (*adequacy*) to meet the level and diversity of need, and research has shown that rural older persons have relatively low *awareness* of the services that do exist in their areas. Available services may also be too costly (*affordability*) for older rural persons. Additional problems can arise in that the services available may not be the ones that are needed (*appropriateness*), something Wallace (1991) has called the "no-care zone." Finally, observers such as Coward (1979) and Rowles (1991) have noted that the content and presentation of the service must fit in with the distinctive attitudes and values found among different rural populations (*acceptability*).

What We Know About Rural Community-Based Services

To date, very little research has been conducted on specific community-based services for rural older persons. In recent work, I have referred to this dearth of information as a "no data zone" (Krout, 1992). Once again we are faced with a gap in what we need in terms of basic and applied research and what is available. We lack simple descriptive data on programs, longitudinal research, and especially programmatic evaluations that look at the short- and long-term impacts of various intervention modalities. Most studies have focused on the availability of various services and have found, not surprisingly, that many individual services are less likely to be available in rural communities.

For example, my own national study of AAAs found that services such as adult day care, respite care, guardianship, material aid, and housing were more likely to be reported as *not available* in rural than in more urban planning and service areas (Krout, 1991d). Rural senior centers generally offer a smaller range of programs as well (Krout, 1989c, 1990b). And statistics on services from AAAs, senior centers, and other agencies probably overstate the actual availability of community-based services to rural older persons, as the services that are available often are less comprehensive and offered less frequently than in urban areas, and are not accessible to all who need them (Krout, 1986). Recently, I noted some generalizations that would appear to characterize the state of community-based services for rural older persons and that can serve as a starting point for this book (Krout, 1992, p. 4):

- Compared with urban elders, rural older persons generally have access to a smaller number and more narrow range of community-based services, especially services for the severely impaired.
- Although the rural-urban service gap has diminished for some services in some areas in the past 20 years, a significant rural disadvantage can still be found.
- Considerable variation is found among rural communities in the richness and diversity of services for older persons, but we know relatively little about the causes of this variation.

- Clear gaps exist in the continuum of care in rural communities. Often there are few alternatives for those who cannot live independently but do not require institutionalization (e.g., community-based services, housing options).
- Too little attention has been given to designing service delivery models and strategies specifically for rural areas and populations. Most rural services are based on programs and policies designed for urban places, and "scaled-down" urban programs have not been shown to be effective. Few service professionals are trained to understand the dynamics of rural communities or know how to plan services for rural populations.
- Little information has been developed or is available to service providers on what program approaches work or do not work in rural communities. Very little evaluation research has been carried out on the impact of various community-based programs on the well-being of rural older persons.
- It has been suggested that rural practitioners face somewhat different challenges and experiences from those faced by urban workers and need different, or additional, skills and knowledge from what are usually provided in most training programs.
- Finally, it is clear that at least some regulatory and reimbursement policies impede the creation, delivery, and survivability of rural community-based services.

These general observations serve as a starting point for the detailed review of individual community-based services that constitutes this book.

Summary and Conclusions

This chapter has provided an overview of the characteristics of rural older populations and the need for community-based services as part of a continuum of care to meet those needs. Overall, the current literature indicates that the community-based services that do exist in rural areas suffer from problems related to availability, accessibility, adequacy, affordability, awareness, acceptability, and appropriateness. More important, a dearth of research and information exists on the planning, development, operation, and effectiveness of current community-based services for older populations. Few descriptions and discussions of alternative programmatic approaches to providing community-based services to the rural elderly are available to assist practitioners and guide policy makers.

Most of the information that has been collected on rural community-based programming is found in local reports or in the files of service providers. Some exceptions to this bleak assessment of the existing knowledge base do exist. The National Resource Center for Rural Elderly (formerly funded by Administration on Aging) has produced close to 20 booklets examining a wide range of services for the rural elderly, and the Center for Rural Aging (funded by the Kellogg Foundation) has collected and assessed a large number of program materials covering rural caregiving, health and wellness promotion, and intergenerational programming. Nonetheless, the information we do have on rural community-based services is far outstripped by what we do not have, and few if any detailed and comprehensive assessments have been attempted that focus on how a wide range of community-based services for rural elders can best be developed and delivered.

The chapters that follow attempt to bring into clearer focus the ways in which various community-based services can be most effectively developed and delivered to rural older persons. The emphasis is on describing and assessing various community-based service approaches and describing the obstacles to providing such services and the programmatic approaches that can overcome them. Obviously, this one book can provide only a starting point for the building of a comprehensive body of research-based literature that provides practitioners and policy makers the guidance they need to refine and improve existing community-based service strategies for older rural populations.

PART II

Service Information, Access, and Coordination

This section comprises four chapters that focus on rural community-based service information, access, and coordination. Although these elements are seen as services in and of themselves, all are also fundamental to the provision of other community-based services for the rural elderly that are examined in subsequent sections of this book.

In Chapter 2, McKinley and Netting present an insightful look at an aspect of providing community-based services that is both ubiquitous and often taken for granted: information and referral. They stress that I&R is the beginning point for any service delivery system and identify a number of assumptions about I&R that are particularly important in any consideration of the service needs of older rural populations. McKinley and Netting identify and review a number of approaches to information and referral in rural areas and discuss the problems that are often encountered in their development and operation, such as the tendency to rely on traditional approaches when creative and unique programs are called for, low rural population density and rural topography and the staff requirements they necessitate, difficulties in maintaining client confidentiality in small communities, and the impact of both in- and out-migration of the old and young on both informal and formal I&R networks. They then discuss what they see as the six core elements of successful rural information and referral systems: the ability to assess needs realistically, understanding of the local community, acknowledgment of rural cultural strengths, acceptance of cultural differences, development of trust among indigenous leaders, and the use of a multimethod approach to service provision. Finally, McKinley and Netting note important research and policy issues for rural information and referral programming.

Chapter 3, by Schauer and Weaver, provides a very comprehensive examination of the transportation needs of rural older persons, with a strong focus on the planning, funding, and operation of rural transportation alternatives. The authors present an overview of how service access problems have increased for the rural elderly in the past decade as a result of demographic, social, and cultural changes; the decline of the rural passenger transportation industry; and the consolidation of rural services in regional centers. They then review and discuss examples of a number of approaches that have been developed to provide transportation assistance to rural elders. These include both informal and formal volunteer services, multiservice providers, and single-purpose transportation agencies based on urban models. A particular strength of the chapter is Schauer and Weaver's clear and concise discussion of the planning- and service-related issues basic to the provision of quality transportation services to rural elders, including appropriate planning methods and tools, service delivery standards, and trained human resources (from drivers to board members). Finally, Schauer and Weaver discuss some of the policy issues that surround this topic. They observe that although highly specialized (and often fragmented) transport systems for specific populations (schoolchildren, disabled persons) are supported in the United States, such support is not nearly as strong for a general rural public transport system. They stress that the role of public-private cooperation in meeting the transport needs of rural elders must be given more attention and support, and that the coordination of existing rural transport must be pushed through stronger legislation at the federal and state levels. Finally, they remind us that greater attention to the mobility needs of rural elders must be explicitly considered in land-use policy and regulation if these needs are to be dealt with holistically and comprehensively.

In Chapter 4, Urv-Wong and McDowell begin by stating that despite the fact that disagreement exists over what the term *case management* means and how the concept is best implemented, commonly accepted goals for this process include assessing the needs of an individual, obtaining appropriate quality services to meet individual needs, and program cost containment. They then discuss the various components of case management in relation to rural practice. Urv-Wong and McDowell continue their insightful analysis with an identification and critique of three rationales they see as often underlying rural case management programs and give particular attention to examining the strengths and weaknesses of activities undertaken in rural areas that are often presented as, but do not in themselves constitute, case management (e.g., service coordination or needs assessment). Their point is that true case management enhances the responsiveness of the existing service system to individual cases through the use of communication and coordination, thereby delivering more to individual clients than could be obtained from discrete services. In the last section of their chapter, Urv-Wong and McDowell present a detailed examination of how general challenges to providing case management, such as definitions, administrative costs, and lack of services and funding, are manifested in rural areas. They also provide some insight into what can be done when rural agencies lack the necessary prerequisites of a case management system and alert us to the important topic of case management standards. Urv-Wong and McDowell pose a fundamental policy issue for rural community-based long-term care systems: Would money spent on case management be more appropriately used to develop comprehensive rural services? They close with a call for more training resources and information to put into practice existing case management guidelines and standards.

Chapter 5, by Krout, Williams, and Owen, provides a useful overview of existing research on rural/urban differences in senior center resources, programming, and participation patterns. Longitudinal data suggest that rural senior centers have not fared as well as their urban counterparts during the 1980s. The authors discuss some of the basic features on which rural senior centers are found to vary, such as facilities, programming, resources and staff, decision-making structure, and focal-point activities. A major focus of the chapter is on identifying and illuminating the basic issues and questions that rural senior center programming must address to be successful: accessibility, affordability, appropriateness, adequacy, and acceptability. The authors also provide a detailed outline of the activities they see as fundamental to operating a rural senior center and present examples of innovative rural senior center approaches to various problems that illustrate the effectiveness of community linkages, aggressive marketing, and creative management. The chapter closes with a discussion of needed research. The authors argue that a lack of consensus on basic policy issues about the roles senior centers should play in the long-term care system, the services they should provide, and who they should serve has created fundamental difficulties and conflicting expectations for these organizations. These and other research, policy, and programming issues need to be resolved if rural senior centers are to reach their full potential as support systems for older persons and as resources for the entire community.

2

Information and Referral

Targeting the Rural Elderly

ANNE H. McKINLEY
F. ELLEN NETTING

Scope, Nature, and Need for I&R

The acronym I&R (for *information and referral*) is common parlance among human service professionals. The term is so taken for granted that we typically use it without thinking about what it means. This chapter examines I&R as a concept. We begin with an examination of definitions, and then explore the historical roots of and basic assumptions about I&R. Next, we focus in turn on the need for I&R among rural elders, on both standard and alternative approaches to I&R, on problems encountered in conducting I&R, and on program needs. We conclude with a discussion of research and policy issues for the provision of I&R to the rural elderly.

Definitions

In 1991 the U.S. Senate Special Committee on Aging asked the U.S. General Accounting Office (GAO) to examine promising approaches to providing I&R. I&R was defined as "the active process of linking someone who has a need or problem with an agency that provides services meeting that need or solving that problem" (Chelimsky, 1991, p. 2).

However, the report quickly acknowledged the limitations of this definition in serving a frail and often vulnerable aged population. Therefore,
some I&R efforts actually evolved into "information and assistance"
(I&A), in which counseling and follow-up are provided (Chelimsky,
1991, p. 14). It is these I&A programs that may offer the most promise
for truly connecting the aged with the services they need.

One can visualize I&R as falling on a continuum that begins with
provision of information only, followed closely by provision of information and referral to an agency, group, or individual. This exchange
would be information and referral in its most elemental form, without
follow-up. In many rural areas, information and referral may become
"information and listening," because isolated individuals may actually
need to use the service person as a sounding board for the venting of
concerns and sharing of frustrations. Next on the continuum one might
envision "information and guidance," which would precede information and assistance as defined above. In short, the range of I&R encompasses a variety of options. In conversations with providers of I&R in
rural areas and in our own experiences we have found the provision of
I&R to be as varied as the persons providing this important service.

Background

Modern I&R systems emerged in both the United Kingdom and the
United States during and after World War II. The British Citizens Advice Bureaus (CABs), largely run by volunteers, provided emergency
information. By 1983 more than 1,000 of these organizations were
operating throughout the British Isles (Levinson, 1988).

In the United States, community advisory centers called Veterans
Information Centers (VICs) were created after World War II. Designed
to aid returning veterans in finding resources, more than 3,000 were
operating throughout the country in 1946. By 1949 the VICs were
closed, most likely because they served only veterans (Levinson, 1988,
p. 17). In the mid-1940s, Chicago established central information centers designed to address chronic disease and long-term care issues. At
the same time, the United Way began to link aging and health resources
through the provision of information.

I&R as a concept was largely a product of the new social programs
of the 1960s, when federal government initiatives promoted the delivery of social services at the local level in both the public and voluntary

sectors. Federal legislation encouraged the development of I&R programs targeting the chronically ill, the mentally ill, and the elderly (Levinson, 1988, pp. 18-19).

Consistent with the development of both voluntary and public agencies in the United States, I&R efforts emerged in both sectors. As federal legislation created I&R services for various target population groups, national voluntary health organizations encouraged I&R program development. For example, in 1913 the American Red Cross used various components of I&R in its home care programs.

I&R was originally considered a high priority for the elderly with the passage of the Older Americans Act in 1965—the Administration on Aging being the only national agency with a federal charge to establish I&R services at local, regional, and state levels (Levinson, 1988, p. 20). I&R, outreach, and transportation services became a trilogy of access services touted as the foundation of the emerging aging network. However, the unique needs and conditions of rural America went largely unrecognized and undefined. In rural counties and towns, fragile community infrastructures and low tax bases did not allow for funding to supplement the minimal dollar allocations for rural program implementation. Neither federal nor state governments were convinced that funding formulas should contain rural designations as a weight factor. At the 1971 White House Conference on Aging, rural areas were finally mentioned specifically in transportation planning, but little change accompanied this recognition.

In the 1970s, the Administration on Aging funded research and a series of working papers that focused on I&R (Levinson, 1988). Virtually all Area Agencies on Aging (AAAs) reported I&R services. They followed no consistent plan, there was little tracking or accountability, and there was no information on program effectiveness adequacy. Furthermore, there was no mention of if or how I&R services responsible to rural areas differed from urban I&R services.

During the 1980s, the aging network began to emphasize direct services, seeing access services such as I&R as only a beginning step. Today, given the increasing complexity of the service delivery system, advocates are calling for a renewed emphasis on I&R, so that older persons and their caregivers can find out how to access services (Chelimsky, 1991, p. 10). This complexity is the result of the increasing fragmentation, specialization, bureaucratization, and competition within the health and human service delivery system.

Assumptions About Rural I&R

In exploring the historical development of I&R, we have identified a number of basic philosophical assumptions. An understanding of these assumptions is important to an understanding of how and why services are delivered to older persons in the United States. It is important to explore the relevance of these assumptions to rural elderly people.

First, I&R is part of all providers' repertoires. It represents the basic communication link between provider and client or between provider and provider. I&R is integral to all settings, across target population groups. I&R is the beginning point for any service delivery system, because prescreening (or screening, intake, or whatever term is used for the first contact a client has with an agency) involves I&R. I&R then is the essential first step in communication that links client with provider. In a sense, then, I&R is an institutionalized part of the service delivery system.

Acknowledging the institutionalized nature of I&R lends itself to immediate questioning by those who live and practice in rural areas. If I&R is institutionalized within the thinking of the formal provider system, what about those geographic areas that are more dependent on informal, neighbor-to-neighbor contact? What happens when rural elders and their families do not know that I&R services exist? How do they find out about them? How do they utilize them to begin a linking process? What happens to rural elders who eventually learn about I&R, call an 800 number, and receive responses from people in a distant town? Perhaps they are given the name of the one agency that can provide them services, but the agency is 40 miles away and has a policy limiting travel to no further than 20 miles to provide the needed service. Has I&R been completed if the referred client is 40 miles away and does not receive the service? Can we then say that I&R is institutionalized in that rural setting?

Second, I&R alone is insufficient in today's system. Without adequate follow-up there is the potential to set up expectations, to deny the potential for older persons to be left in a system that "passes the buck," and essentially to do harm to the very persons the system should be designed to serve. Without follow-up I&R is meaningless, because we cannot evaluate what occurs. Therefore, *information and assistance* may be the more appropriate terminology, and I&R may be outdated language. It is important to note, however, that just because I&A may be more ideal than I&R does not mean that it would be any easier to evaluate. In rural areas where available staff are limited, outside assistance may be required, thus creating barriers to the evaluation process. Persons or organizations from outside the community who may become involved in planning, monitoring, and evaluating I&R services in rural areas must give careful consideration and sensitive attention to community profiles and take the time to gain a working knowledge of local policies and procedures. Extra funding as well as staff may be limited and thus increase barriers to a monitoring and evaluation process that is difficult—and may even be impossible—to breach.

Third, I&R occurs interorganizationally (across organizations) and intraorganizationally (between programs and services within the same organization). In other words, I&R is not just a linkage mechanism between client and provider but serves as the basic communication link between provider and provider. These linkages are the essence of what we call *networking*. For example, in large bureaucracies with multiple units delivering services to various constituencies, I&R has become a way of life. How many providers have asked for information and assistance within their own organizations, whether they need to know who has been hired to replace the coordinator of the home health program or where a client goes to locate services beyond their agency? I&R is the glue that connects questions to appropriate answers. If the answers are not forthcoming, one is unable to move forward. In rural areas, where there are fewer freestanding providers and where the agencies that do exist may be satellites of a larger bureaucracy, the information is frequently late in arriving. When it does arrive, the interpretation from a metropolitan center may not fit the local cultural environment, further complicating forward movement and progress for both worker and client.

Fourth, just as the Omnibus Reconciliation Act mandates of 1987 led to a rediscovery of the importance of nurses' aides in long-term care facilities, it is time to rediscover the incredibly critical role played by designated persons who provide I&R. These persons are often secretaries and receptionists who are tied to their desks, answering questions all day. They may not be highly trained professionals, but what they do can make the difference in whether an older client pursues a task or gives up in hopelessness. These persons have to think on their feet, respond to unpredictable requests, demonstrate active listening skills, interpret what is really needed, and know what is being requested. Without sensitive I&R personnel, clients can be further disempowered and disenfranchised. With sensitive personnel, clients may find hope and support.

Fifth, to empower clients, I&R providers have to know how to span boundaries and how to conceptualize beyond those boundaries. Creativity is essential, because clients' requests will not always link up directly with available services. The I&R employee responsible for giving information needs to know and understand that callers may not know how to ask for what they need or how to describe their problems. Consequently, recognition of key words and phrases becomes part of the conceptualization of boundaries. In rural areas it is critical to recognize real boundaries, perceived boundaries, and created boundaries. Recognizing when clients resist going beyond geographic boundaries is also essential. Cultural and ethnic diversity in rural areas may dictate where people are willing to go to receive services and from whom they are willing to accept help.

The need for creativity in I&R provision is illustrated by one recent case in which an I&R person answered the phone to hear a distraught caregiver ask how she could get her invalid mother's hair done. She lived several miles from the nearest hairdresser and her mother did not feel like traveling over bumpy country roads. The I&R worker knew that beautician services were not offered in the "aging network," but she happened to think of a beautician who had offered to go to the homes of older persons in neighboring rural communities. This referral was a creative response to an atypical request. The beautician was as important to the aging network as any other helping professional, because she was able to provide a service to fill an identified need.

Sixth, case management has emerged out of the basic need for usable information, referral, and assistance. If one views case management as a process of assessing needs and translating those needs into care planning, I&R could be viewed as a shortened version of that translation. If one sees case management as part of a feedback system in which clients receive services and then how the services worked for them is evaluated, then essentially this is the "assistance" that we hope I&R will incorporate. Case management can then be seen as a logical extension of an information and referral system.

An I&R system model with steps that involve triaging into levels of care illustrates this sixth assumption. Level 1 in this model is the client who is able to take and use information without further assistance. This could be by telephone or through an educational seminar, a brochure, or a workshop. Level 2 is the client who needs assistance in linking with an agency. This could include making telephone connection or counseling to develop a plan, with little assistance beyond that. In Level 3 the client needs full case management planning with extensive monitoring and assistance. Level 4 would be return of a client to independent functioning, better informed and able to access the I&R system should new needs arise. This program model allows a client to enter the system through I&R at any point of need, to be maintained in the system at a determined level of care, or to be terminated from the system having regained independence. Two systems utilizing variations of this model are Missouri's Enriched I&R and a step-up case management system devised in a rural Arizona hospital (McKinley & Peterson, 1988).

Seventh, there is an assumption that all who develop needs that cannot be met by their existing social systems should have I&R access. Persons should know where they can go for help if they should need it. Prevention is a large part of I&R's purpose, and if people know where to go for help they can circumvent crisis care. This would be a desirable goal for rural seniors and their families.

One of the authors directed a rural senior citizens' center in a small eastern Tennessee county. There were many retired persons in this county, many of whom had no intention of coming to the center for planned activities. They felt that "others" probably needed this kind of "help," but they were very willing to assist in fund-raising for the center or in renovating the old building so that "others" could use it. As they aged and developed needs, however, they knew who to call in their rural community to locate resources. They called the senior center director, who was responsible for I&R. In short, many well elderly in rural areas may never feel the need to call, but if they know who to call when a need arises, they can access services through I&R.

Last, people often assume that anyone can do I&R in rural areas. Therefore, we may have missed an opportunity to examine the essential ingredients of what happens in the day-to-day contacts made by thousands of I&R workers who listen to the requests of older persons and their caregivers in nonurban areas. How to approach these encounters in rural areas is what this chapter is all about.

Need for I&R Among Rural Elders

Rural elders in the United States have many of the same needs and problems encountered by their urban counterparts. The differences between the two groups are found in degree of need, with rural elderly having "less income, poorer health, inferior housing, and . . . access to less adequate transportation systems" (Krout, 1989a, p. 3). Combined with this greater need are resource problems. Rural areas do not have the constellation of formal services available in urban areas. This is not surprising, given the geographic distances and limited transportation systems in many rural environments (Krout, 1989a). Therefore, I&R may be more difficult to provide in rural areas because appropriate referrals can be made only when services are available. I&R providers in rural areas must continually devise new methods to maximize limited resources and in some cases may be painfully aware of needs that simply cannot be met in their communities.

Rural areas are frequently dependent on public funding to develop services. A low population base does not provide a lucrative or profitable environment for private entrepreneurial effort, so private funding is often not available. Therefore, funding I&R programs, as well as other services, is problematic for rural providers.

Given these limited resources, what happens to rural people in need of service? How do they solve critical service needs? Do I&R systems play a part in problem resolution? If I&R is viewed solely as a formally funded and formally organized system, probably not. If I&R is envisioned as a neighbor-to-neighbor, informal system, probably so. This type of information sharing is a critical ingredient to rural people and their communities. It is no less viable than the more sophisticated methods used in urban areas, and is in far greater danger of becoming extinct without moral support and technical assistance that could be provided at low cost by formally structured organizations. In broadening the vision and thinking about I&R for rural areas, it is necessary to determine whether I&R is only "inreach" (people calling for help in a situation of immediate importance for "fixing"), whether it is also "outreach" (people receiving information for planning before a need arises), or whether it includes elements of each.

Whether it has elements of each is relevant to the situation of Mary and Russell, a couple who are lifetime residents in an area that is extremely rural and meets guidelines for frontier living (six people per square mile, according to the U.S. Department of the Interior). They live below the poverty level in a house that needs insulation, plumbing, and electrical repairs. Russell worked for a short time after World War II in a manufacturing job before returning to farming. Mary has been a housewife all of her married life. The couple calls an 800 I&R number (which they heard about at the local post office) to get nursing home information for Russell's mother, who has lived with them for the past five years. What they don't ask about are home repair, food stamps, medical information for themselves, commodities, and SSI benefits, even though they would be eligible for all of these services. They don't know to ask—they don't know these services are available, and they don't know they're eligible. In many 800 number models, only the nursing home question would be answered. Does the I&R provider have a responsibility to give other information? Is there a way for the I&R provider to know that there is other valuable information that could enhance quality of life for Russell and Mary? These are questions for policy, for practice, and for ethical consideration in the development of rural I&R programs.

Standard and Alternative Approaches to Rural I&R

Standard Approaches

Given the emergence of I&R across settings and populations over the past few decades, modes of providing this service have varied extensively. In 1972, the Alliance of Information and Referral Systems (AIRS) was given birth by the National Conference on Social Welfare. In 1978, AIRS held its first national conference. AIRS membership has expanded over the years, and its members are linked through local chapter development, newsletters, journals, and studies related to I&R (Levinson, 1988).

In 1983, the Administration on Aging established a consortium to promote information linkages across organizations within communities and to promote networking among I&R providers. This consortium included such disparate groups as AIRS, the United Way of America, the U.S. Army, and AT&T. That same year, AIRS and the United Way of America issued the first set of *National Standards for Information and Referral* (AIRS, 1983). Development of model standards was supported by an Administration on Aging grant (Levinson, 1988).

In 1991, the National Information and Referral Support Center, a joint project of the National Association of State Units on Aging, AIRS, and the National Association of Area Agencies on Aging developed national standards for I&R services funded under the Older Americans Act. Citing the lack of a uniform reporting system as problematic for obtaining data on what happens within the aging network, these standards attempt to guide service system development. Two components make up this I&R initiative: (a) the National I&R Training and Technical

Support Center, designed to "support qualitative improvements in I&R design, management, operations, and staff development," including standards development; and (b) the National I&R Locator Service, created to "enhance the visibility of I&R services among older people and [to] operate and promote a national 800 number to link consumers to the appropriate state and local I&R service" (Chelimsky, 1991, p. 11).

Standards can be viewed as minimal guidelines that establish basic expectations for what will happen. We will not reiterate these standards here because they are readily available through the National Information and Referral Support Center. Our purpose is to delve into the intricacies of how one actually faces the I&R challenge in rural areas so that standards are upheld and depth is achieved.

Alternative Approaches

A number of books explain in detail how to develop I&R systems. Mathews and Fawcett (1981) provide a practical overview of how to develop an I&R system, how to provide the service, and checks to use in quality oversight. They take the reader from the point of gathering community information and organizing a social service directory to the development of forms to be used at each step of the process. In 1984, Levinson and Haynes edited *Accessing Human Services: International Perspectives,* which provides insight into I&R models developed around the world. This volume contains 14 reports from nine countries. Although the strategies and structures for developing access systems vary tremendously, Levinson and Haynes (1984) indicate that the basic purpose of these systems is to link individuals with the most accessible services available. Levinson also has developed an insightful overview titled *Information and Referral Networks,* published in 1988. This volume provides excellent information on how to organize I&R systems and looks at megatrends for the future. Levinson sees I&R as having great potential, although she describes it as "embryonic and uneven" (p. 185).

Although I&R is most likely targeted to those persons considered vulnerable through frailty or isolation, we believe that I&R should be available to all persons. Therefore, it is incumbent upon us to discuss I&R in the context of outreach. "Outreach takes the services of information and referral out of an agency or center into the community" (Steun, 1985, p. 88). However, "if outreach is undertaken, it is important to be able to respond positively to requests for service" (p. 89). This is the basic dilemma faced by I&R programs in rural communities. It is important to let older persons know the aging network is in the community, but it is also important that they understand the limitations in addressing all the existing needs.

Common approaches to outreach include personal in-home visits; telephone calls; correspondence and printed materials, including handouts, flyers, and brochures; development of service directories; hot lines and toll-free numbers; radio and television spots; and the use of volunteers (Steun, 1985). These methods are often used to get the word out and to encourage older persons to seek assistance.

This is when I&R providers begin to look across boundaries and to think creatively, with citizens and consumers as participants in the process. Steun (1985) urges us to rethink outreach and to search for nontraditional approaches to reaching the elderly. Possibly, a provider needs to reconceptualize the service delivery system. For example, county or small town officials and their staffs may be the first point of contact for some older persons. County supervisors in a rural county may know many of those in the older population well, and they can assist in informing them about what services are available and where to go for help. Using an arrangement such as that for emergency assistance numbers (911) or looking at cooperative partnerships with places where 911 exists may be an option in some rural communities. Emergency medical people, rural fire departments, and sheriff's departments provide satellite offices that are nontraditional partners for many more providers and not a "first thought" for people needing information.

Similarly, rural health clinics and hospitals are visited by older persons more than by any other group. Aging network staff have every reason to connect with discharge planners in rural or regional medical centers, because they are being forced to discharge older patients into communities that do not always have needed long-term care services. Public utilities often publish newsletters or are willing to put flyers in with monthly billing statements. Religious groups, parish nurse networks, farm organizations, schools, colleges, regional shopping complexes, agriculture extension systems, post offices, and small businesses are features of the rural landscape that take on great significance in small communities.

Conceptualizing the aging network as any linkage to older persons through all available groups and organizations in rural communities may open up new possibilities. For example, a local SSI targeting program in Arizona found that elementary schools were appropriate locations for identifying low-income older persons. Children who qualified for a subsidized lunch program often had grandparents who were struggling to make ends meet.

Methods of outreach will vary by community, and the I&R provider must understand the culture of an individual community before assuming that any one method will work. Multiple methods in different arrangements will work for specific communities. Word of mouth is probably the most effective way to get information out, and radio shows can span broad distances. Identifying a core of indigenous community leaders who will serve as an advisory group may be a way to begin. If the rural community has a senior center, this may serve as the hub for I&R. Centers may be designated focal points for the aging network. These traditional avenues of service delivery must be connected with the more nontraditional organizations mentioned above if I&R is going to be effective. Although research shows that 90% of centers say they do I&R (Krout, 1989a), there are few tracking and accountability systems to define what this includes and to determine levels of effectiveness. It is also important to recognize that many rural communities do not have senior centers, and that, when they do, there may be a select group of attendees. This select group may be determined by variables such as transportation availability, cultural and social stratification, interest, and economics.

One must be careful not to make assumptions about how outreach efforts will contribute to increased I&R calls. Calsyn (1989) reports the implementation of an outreach effort called the Carrier Alert Program. Designed to reach isolated rural elders, the project used letter carriers, fraternal organizations, clergy, and home extension agents to assist in case finding. Calsyn indicates that the program did not work as well as expected, for two reasons. First, the potential referral agents may not have been as committed as they needed to be, having other social causes in which they were also engaged. The lesson learned was that it would be wise to spend more time in reminding the agents to be on the lookout for the elderly who were in most need (i.e., economically deprived, socially isolated, health care risks, minorities). Second, there were attitudinal barriers on the part of some rural people who were reluctant to use government services. However, Calsyn points out that the elderly in this county were often in great need because younger support persons had left the community to seek employment in more urban areas. This left many of these persons without adequate community supports. Calsyn concludes that "letter carriers may offer the most promise in helping service providers identify needy elderly [because they] have the potential for daily contact with the elderly" (p. 133).

Other programs with similar features are the "gatekeeper" programs developed and implemented by Ray Raschko (1990) in Spokane, Washington, and other outreach gatekeeper programs described by Lorraine Lidoff (1984). These programs utilize utility workers, store clerks, and others in small towns who frequently see local residents.

A 1991 GAO study asked respondents to identify the I&R program features that would contribute to promising practice. Four categories were identified:

- locating I&R services where elderly populations live or frequently visit
- hiring professional staff, including minorities, to serve diverse cultural populations
- using automated information resources and telephone technology to provide information effectively
- publicizing I&R to the elderly and their caregivers through active outreach methods (Chelimsky, 1991, p. 13)

On paper, these program features read well. In rural areas, however, I&R providers must consider the feasibility of implementing systems that are dependent upon electronic technology, even telephones. Flexibility in program design and potential funding must allow for innovative interpretations by and for rural people. Rural formal and informal networks may not be able to apply high-tech methods because of staffing definitions or equipment requirements.

Problems Encountered in Providing Rural I&R

Restraining and Driving Forces

A number of restraining forces must be considered by those providing I&R in rural areas. First, providers who have limited opportunity to share ideas can become tied to manuals and standard approaches. In times when financial resources are limited and staff are stretched thin, it is essential to think of and provide new, alternative approaches to I&R and outreach.

It is important to meet with other providers, to evaluate what is and is not being done and to share and use ideas. In rural areas where there

are few service providers and each has a specifically targeted population, it is helpful to combine efforts to get information out. Although
this effort may invite early turf battles, it can begin a linking that is
profitable to the providers in terms of money, time, and energy.

Second, sheer geographic distances are a major consideration in rural
areas. If I&R is to include outreach as well as "inreach," providers must
remember how diverse rural communities are. What is rural for eastern
Tennessee, for example, seems much less rural than the area found in
traveling the Navajo Reservation in Arizona. Not only are factors such
as climate and road accessibility of extreme importance in the planning
of outreach efforts, but lack of transportation to span those spaces may
be equally problematic.

Third, staff and volunteer time is precious. Conducting in-home visits
takes on an entirely different meaning when travel time between homes
is measured in hours rather than minutes. When volunteers are used to
provide services, they must be carefully recruited, trained, and super-
vised. Their efforts must be recognized, and they must be encouraged
to become part of a team. In addition, they must be sensitive to the
diverse cultural perspectives they encounter.

A fourth restraining force comes from the difficulty of respecting
privacy and maintaining confidentiality. This is particularly problematic in those rural communities where people know one another well.
Indigenous volunteers and staff have to be trained to understand that
sharing information (a basic norm in many communities) is different
when that information is obtained as part of their paid or volunteer
involvement in a formally structured I&R program. The client, too, has
to be reassured and prepared when volunteers are used.

Fifth, migration affects planning, development, and delivery of I&R
and other services. The out-migration of the young and the young-old
from rural areas is a potential impediment to the availability of informal
I&R sources. In some rural retirement areas with significant seasonal
out- and in-migration, there may be difficulties in maintaining informal
supports as healthy and economically secure persons may leave and the
ill and poor remain.

The restraining forces discussed above were documented in two community organization programs that were designed for rural communities
in a rural 9,000-square-mile county in Arizona (see McKinley & Goodman, 1984). In one program a community volunteer auxiliary provides
I&R. In the other, an organization for combined informal services has
formed. A common theme is the provision of ongoing consultation,

in-service, and technical assistance from a formal structure that in the first instance was 60 miles away and in the second instance 45 miles away.

Before I&R providers throw up their hands in despair, it is also important for them to recognize driving or motivating forces. First, it has been our experience that many of those persons who constitute the aging network are creative individuals who want to make changes happen. Pooling this creative energy has great potential.

Second, the development of a strengths perspective is helpful. Often, the rural elderly are discussed from the perspective that they are "worse off" than their urban counterparts. Ironically, such a view may miss the strengths the rural elderly bring to the aging network because it concentrates on problems. Stamina in dealing with vast geographic distances, strength in facing barriers, and experience in dealing with separation and isolation may be resources often overlooked.

Third, rural areas allow providers to take a more individualized approach to I&R. What works for one subgroup in the community may not attract others. The crowding and the demands perpetrated on the formal delivery system that occur in more urban areas are nonexistent.

Core Elements of Successful Rural Approaches

There are a number of core elements to be found in successful I&R and outreach in rural communities. First is the ability to assess needs realistically. It is important that providers engage older persons and their families in network building, but this is complicated in rural areas by transportation over great distances and unpredictable communication resources. One aspect of building any network is to hear what the needs are—not just the demands that reach provider agencies, but those needs that have not reached the doorway of a service system. Reaching out so that persons make their needs known means that the I&R provider becomes a source of valuable needs data. The I&R provider, armed with the data, has the opportunity to work on prioritizing needs, setting short- and long-term goals, interpreting progress and direction, and helping people in the area understand and participate in the process.

Second, understanding the local community is essential. This means beginning with an adequate sociodemographic community profile. This is necessary whether I&R is provided in a highly concentrated or geographically dispersed environment. However, in rural communities the smaller population base can allow factions to emerge that present deep schisms based on individual personalities. There is less anonymity and more chance for daily encounters. This can be confronted successfully if the I&R provider maintains neutrality.

Third, understanding the community means acknowledging cultural strengths, those communal experiences that give the people combined goals, loyalties, and identity. No two rural communities are alike, and cultural strengths come from years of coping in diverse environments. It is essential for professionals to listen to the people who live in rural communities and to reach agreement with residents to provide support and to consult (if necessary), but not to replace what people want. The role of the provider is to use professional knowledge and experience to aid in refining definitions of need and to offer support and guidance that can lead to successful I&R implementation.

Fourth, once cultural strengths are acknowledged, the provider must learn to accept that there are differences. It is not up to the I&R service provider to change culture or to embrace a particular way of looking at life. Providers must be sensitive to ethnic diversity, language, and cultural differences. It is up to the provider, however, to accept the differences and to provide service that respects these differences.

Fifth, trust must develop or I&R will not be utilized. This means that I&R providers must give information that is usable and reliable. This does not mean that there will always be an answer to every question, but that there is a commitment to facing each challenge in a sensitive and caring manner. Trust emanates from a network of indigenous leaders as staff, volunteers, and influentials who have a shared vision of what can work in a rural community.

Sixth, the I&R system must be built on a multimethod approach to service provision. Once the provider knows and understands the community, it will be up to a committed group of persons to employ those strategies that they believe will work, given the diversity within that rural community. No two communities will be the same.

Rural I&R Program Needs

The above discussion leads to three basic program needs for developing I&R services in rural communities. Each is discussed below, with appropriate illustrations.

First, there is a need for system development. Various sources cited in this chapter identify different ways to develop an I&R system. However, it is essential that leaders in the rural community be open to the changes that professionals want to put into place. It is equally important that professionals be responsive to the needs identified by community members, both interested citizens and consumers of service. Ownership is particularly important, because rural communities may comprise people who know one another quite well. However, it is important that providers not assume automatically that people in rural communities know one another.

A complicating factor in system development is that I&R will not work without adequate resources in the local community or in close proximity. The I&R point of entry becomes crucial, then, because it may also become the hub of activity where unmet needs are identified. Methods of identifying and documenting unmet needs are mandatory if these needs are to be addressed and recognized. Otherwise, the I&R center becomes a place where people find out that they have to leave their community of origin in order to locate the services they need in their old age.

Second, there is a crying need for orientation to the I&R mission, staff development, and ongoing training. Ideal training for I&R begins with the hiring process. Personnel who have an inherent sensitivity to people in need or under stress are required. Desired characteristics include excellent communication skills, an understanding of aging, an understanding of behaviors that accompany chronic illness, ability to apply methods of handling personal frustrations, ability to handle difficult callers, assertiveness, and listening skills. Staff need to be open to new methods and alternative approaches in order to continue outreach efforts. They must be able to work closely with, recruit, and supervise volunteers. Community building is a part of the development of an I&R system in rural communities.

Third, sensitivity to diverse client groups with differing needs is crucial. I&R efforts and outreach methods must be compatible. There must be consistent and regular updating of resources, including service location, telephone numbers, available services, eligibility guidelines, and target populations. Available resources include nonprofit, for-profit, and public providers as well as informed groups and associations.

Research and Policy Issues

The Administration on Aging has made progress in encouraging the development of standards and in advocating for a more uniform reporting system. This process needs to continue. Currently, I&R programs do not always collect comparable data. In some rural areas, I&R programs do not collect enough information to report what is happening and to document requested needs that cannot be met. Without this information, decision makers may not be convinced that limited resources should be used to address these needs. A minimum set of research questions would center on documentation of requests, needs met, and needs unmet. The data would begin to develop a picture of whether I&R is a usable, useful program in rural America. The data would assist rural advocates in applying for program development and operation monies. More broadly, researchers might begin to answer the question of whether I&R as originally named and envisioned continues to be a viable concept.

With the current emphasis on client outcomes, it is important to ask what clients consider to be a successful I&R intervention. Once basic descriptive data are available, I&R programs need to determine what outcomes are important to measure, and these outcomes need to be client centered. Studies indicate that rural elderly persons rely more heavily upon informal systems than do their urban counterparts (Dwyer, Lee, & Coward, 1990). The question is whether this is by choice or out of necessity. Studies that focus on the choices, preferences, expectations, and utilization of services by rural elderly will inform our understanding of what outcomes I&R networks need to address.

Research is needed on the actual process of I&R provision—focusing on rural practice and what works there. Rural practitioners, planners, and policy makers need to understand better the impact of fragmented communication and "noncommunication" systems, how informal networks are used and the effectiveness or lack of effectiveness of urban, centralized numbers, other technologies, and different approaches.

Policy

Several policy questions are raised by this discussion. First, should I&R and outreach be mandated when requesters cannot be referred because services are not available? In other words, does this set up expectations and hopes that are rapidly dashed in rural areas? This is not only a policy issue, but a basic ethical dilemma. If I&R locations become the hubs for identifying requests that cannot be met in the elderly person's environment, then there is a responsibility to address those requests.

Second, how can services be better targeted to the rural elderly? Policies must be flexible so that diversity among the rural aged is respected. Policy makers need to address "rural solutions" rather than assume that the replication of urban methods will translate to rural areas. Some methods will, but others may not.

Third, there are policy issues surrounding the allocation of funding. How will distribution of funds be decided? How will equity of I&R programs be achieved when the primary considerations are for high-density populations? Although there are areas designated as rural in which ethnic minorities make up a high percentage of the population and need special consideration in funding, there are many rural areas that are penalized in the funding process because their percentages of ethnic minorities are low.

Fourth, planners and policy makers need insight into how rural providers and people feel about information given and services rendered. Frequently in rural areas, providers seem to react more negatively and intensely to the lack of available information and services because of their great awareness of the vastness of the need. People in rural areas may see only their own plight, and may begin to feel powerless to change their situation. Therefore it is imperative that decision makers have mechanisms in place so that the voices of rural America can be heard.

Summary and Conclusions

This chapter has taken a broad, in-depth look at I&R as a concept, a statement of policy, and a service program. I&R may seem to be a straightforward concept, but it is complex to implement, especially so in a rural context. The literature exploring the importance of I&R is limited, yet this is a program component that is so much a part of the human delivery system that it is taken for granted. In rural areas, I&R program design and implementation tend to be as diverse as the communities served and are sometimes nonexistent.

Realizing the potential of I&R requires imagination and creativity that transcend "rural fatigue." Recalling the power of information and the relief of knowing where to go for help can motivate both provider and consumer. In an atmosphere that continues to emphasize direct service, the access trilogy (I&R, outreach, and transportation) needs to be reviewed—perhaps given a new name or shifted in its direction.

3

Rural Elder Transportation

PETER M. SCHAUER
PATRICIA WEAVER

In the array of services necessary to sustain independent living for elders in rural America, transportation is distinct in its role of providing access to all other life activities. Virtually no other services are attainable without transportation. Conditions unique to rural areas are particularly damaging to the ability of the social network to serve needs of the elderly: isolation, limited availability of resources, services and facilities that are widely dispersed, poor condition of rural roads, and rising costs (Bell & Revis, 1983; Kaiser, 1991; Youmans, 1980).

An adequate, well-publicized transportation system is particularly critical to rural elders, whose access to the network may be limited by physical abilities, economics, or personal choice. Their need for transportation is as great as that of their urban counterparts, and the need continues to grow as these individuals grow older (Kaiser, 1991). However, even though the need is great, elders with limited experience with modes of transportation other than the private automobile are resistant to major changes in their travel behavior and are more likely to rely on learning about travel options from friends and relatives (Sperling & Goralka, 1988). The ways in which rural elders are encouraged to use transportation may be as critical as the actual availability of services.

Critical elements in a transportation network include means by which individuals are transported, either intracommunity or intercommunity, for a variety of essential and discretionary services; means by which goods and services are delivered to and exported from the community; and an adequate infrastructure upon which to deliver these services. The integrity of the rural transportation network has been assaulted and fragmented continuously over the past 30 years. The challenge to policy makers and planners to develop strategies by which to finance and maintain at least a minimum level of essential services has been significant and often neglected.

The specific task for policy makers and practitioners alike is to identify the special travel needs of rural elders and to identify approaches that individuals and communities may use to meet these needs. Some rural communities have been successful in implementing innovative service designs and may provide guidance to other communities striving to develop appropriate systems or to enhance existing services.

Background

In the post-World War II era in the United States, resources were allocated on a disproportional basis to interstate highway construction, a highway network that runs through less than one-third of the nonmetropolitan counties in the United States (Walzer & Chicoine, 1989). During this period of intensive interstate highway construction to connect urban areas of the United States, public resources were directed to the once privately operated urban passenger transportation system to ensure its survival. National priorities were focused on meeting needs of urban intracity transportation and intercity transportation connecting urbanized areas, with no prevailing public policy to meet or protect intrarural access needs.

It was not until the War on Poverty era of the 1960s, with its emphasis on rural social services development, that local planners recognized mobility, even with an adequate infrastructure, as a problem. In the post-interstate construction era, many states began to discover that they could not construct their way out of congestion. The rural mobility problem has worsened over the past decade because of special demographic, social, and cultural aspects of rural mobility; the distribution of rural services; and the general decline of the formal and informal rural passenger transportation network.

Demographic, Social, and Cultural Changes
Affecting Rural Elder Mobility

The number of elderly unable to drive for reasons of health or poverty has increased at the same time that rural passenger transportation has deteriorated. A greater proportion of elderly live in rural areas, with growing numbers of elderly over age 75 who are unable to drive or who have limited driving ability. Their access to medical care, social services, and their own communities is generally inadequate.

In addition to changes in rural demographic patterns, there are subgroups of elderly who have particular need for special transportation, such as Native Americans living on reservations, migrant families, rural poor elderly, and frail elderly with physical disabilities. Each group has special service considerations, but transportation delivery schemes have not always recognized the unique needs of these populations.

Although special transportation systems have been developed, some elderly meet their mobility needs through their families. Transportation to the doctor, shopping, or other necessary transportation services provided by relatives may represent opportunities for interaction between the elderly person and family members. At the opposite extreme, elders may avoid family-provided transportation because it threatens their sense of independence or excessively burdens their relationship with relatives who can drive (National Eldercare Institute on Transportation, 1992a). Others may choose travel modes other than the family because they recognize that their relatives' economic survival depends on an uninterrupted presence at work that may be compromised by the need to provide for the transportation of an older family member.

In most rural areas the family is no longer the transportation option that it once was, given the dispersion of youth to urban areas where jobs and other opportunities exist. Kaiser (1991) found that "rural nonfarm elderly are the least likely to have proximate children," affording less opportunity to rely on family members for transportation. Although these individuals may utilize a network of friends and neighbors for transportation, many are reluctant to impose. Additionally, the transportation options of friends and neighbors in communities where the elderly population exceeds 25% of the total may be just as limited. Without the ability to drive or to access other formal or informal transportation options, the rural elder is truly isolated.

Decline of the Rural Passenger Transportation Industry

The decline of the passenger transportation industry in rural areas represents one of the most significant challenges to mobility for rural elders. The Bus Regulatory Reform Act of 1982 deregulated the bus industry, and by 1986 it is estimated that more than 4,500 service points had been lost, with a majority occurring in communities with populations of 10,000 or below (U.S. Department of Agriculture, 1989, p. 13). Today, residents of most rural communities not traversed by an interstate highway rarely are able to utilize intercity bus services.

Although the decline of the intercity bus industry has been symptomatic of the general increase in difficulty of access and mobility for the rural elderly, it is by no means the only rural access and mobility problem. Lack of adequate emergency transportation for health care, limited or nonexistent local taxi service, poor availability of long-distance rail or air service, and lack of transportation service during nonbusiness hours are also major problems.

Distribution of Rural Services

In the past 20 years the United States has experienced phenomenal growth in the number of vehicle miles traveled, and Americans are considerably more mobile than they were in 1960. In 1983, the average distance traveled by an individual in the United States was approximately 8,500 miles; distance traveled by an individual over age 65 was only about half that amount (Duensing, 1988). The increase in vehicle miles traveled corresponds with the decentralization of most American cities and small towns; even residents of rural areas find that travel to dispersed locations is more necessary than before. The consolidation of medical services, dispersion of services throughout the community, and decline of the central business district in small towns represent just three of the critical factors challenging access in rural areas. Increasing reliance on the private auto has made it difficult to sustain a broad-based mass transportation system; those who cannot use private automobiles become more isolated.

The distribution of shopping, health, and social services in communities has special impact on the provision of transportation. Even very small rural communities have become polycentric, losing their central business districts to strip malls and shops where automobiles can park with relative ease. When new services are developed in areas outside the central business district and away from the community's principal activity areas, walking to the services is difficult and increases the miles of travel required to meet daily living needs. Trip generators are dispersed, and providing mass transportation service is more difficult.

The lack of rural human service infrastructure is particularly noticeable in the health care field. Many rural hospitals are moving toward the provision of primary care in non-acute care situations only (Teigen, 1991). A "hub-and-spoke" service pattern is developing, with growing numbers of patients from smaller hospitals referred to larger hospitals in regional and metropolitan areas. The implication for rural services is that vehicles committed outside the local area to travel to regional hospitals cannot provide service to local shopping, nutrition sites, doctors, or other local transportation needs.

Long-distance medical trips are especially difficult to schedule. Often the vehicle must leave early in the morning and cannot return until late afternoon. Other riders may not find the long trip compatible with shopping or other nonmedical trips; consequently, coordinated ridership levels are low. As rural hospitals are consolidated, the need for transportation for non-acute care purposes will increase, especially for the elderly who do not wish to drive to regional centers or who feel uncomfortable driving in metropolitan areas.

Hospitals typically provide rural health care in one of two ways: Services are offered in mobile units, with roving or circuit-rider physicians, or clinics are established in rural areas. The usual scenario is to provide health care from a regional hospital, to which the individual is transported for services. The hub-and-spoke transportation system serving the regional hospitals, operated either by the hospital or by a regional transportation service, is essential when private automobile transportation is unavailable.

With the lack of widely available rural human services, it is clear that the low population densities in rural areas relative to urban areas represents a low demand yet high need for public transportation services. *Demand* is presented as an economic concept: the amount of service people are willing to purchase at a given price. *Need* refers to the social consequences of not providing transportation and is difficult to measure in any precise way. In a sparsely populated rural area where there are few shopping opportunities, health services, and social services, the willingness or ability to pay for public transportation is low. However, public policy developed since the late 1970s has recognized the need for transportation of individuals to services, despite the low demand. Transportation investment has been determined to be worthwhile and essential for delivery of services to those in rural areas with socially defined needs.

Approaches to Elder Mobility: Typical Service Delivery in the Rural United States

Rural areas cannot be described in terms of homogeneous characteristics; likewise, transportation services in rural areas are available along a full continuum of complexity and level of service. Approaches to elder mobility range from volunteer driver networks using personal vehicles to highly organized multiservice providers and single-purpose providers modeled on urban transit authorities.

Volunteer Services

Volunteer networks traditionally have been one of the most prevalent forms of passenger transportation in rural areas. Volunteer service is used extensively in both informal and formal networks sponsored by churches or other social service organizations. It is not uncommon for family and friends to transport neighbors at no cost or for modest fees that may be intended as small token payments or for larger payments intended to compensate for vehicle wear and tear and some of the driver's time.

Church-related activities are among the most important discretionary travel trips taken by rural elders, yet transportation to such activities is the service least likely to be available from more formal transportation providers (Kaiser, 1991). However, churches often organize volunteer networks for their parishioners, offering elders a way to maintain or sustain their spiritual and social lives in a rural community. In addition to church-related transportation, senior center outreach programs may provide transportation through a network of senior drivers. Senior centers usually focus their efforts on nutrition and shopping activities, but in many low population density areas the services provided by senior centers or religious organizations are the only transportation services available for those without cars.

A more formally organized volunteer program in a rural area will include screening of volunteer drivers, vehicle inspections, and reimbursement for mileage for transporting individuals. These types of services are especially useful for the one-person medical trip, particularly when the individual must travel a long distance or needs an assistant. One of the most innovative volunteer services is conducted in Mercer County, West Virginia, where individuals are provided with automobiles; in turn, individuals provided with cars are responsible for transporting others. In another program in southeast Kansas, four communities share a vehicle that is passed from one community to the next each day of the week; a volunteer driver in each community operates the vehicle for that day much like a taxicab, providing transportation to those in the community who need it. A program in five rural communities near Lafayette, Indiana, provides more than 15,000 trips per year with five vans operated by volunteer drivers. These drivers receive extensive training, the same as paid employees would receive (National Eldercare Institute on Transportation, 1992a).

Multiservice Agencies

More organized rural service providers provide passenger transportation through a menu of social service activities, such as nutrition services, adult day care, and job services, using small vans or minibuses. Community action programs, Area Agencies on Aging, Councils on Aging, senior center and nutrition programs, and health departments often provide small vans or small buses for transporting individuals to their programs.

Eagle Transit in Kalispell, Montana, a transportation service sponsored by the Council on Aging, has developed a brokerage system in which several transportation services are available, ranging from taxis to minibuses (Weaver, Schauer, Proctor, & Day, 1991, Appendix B). Florida has initiated a program in which school buses can be utilized for transportation of senior citizens during times when they are not used by schoolchildren.

Single-Purpose Transportation Agencies

The second most common model of service provision is a single-purpose transportation service provider. The single-purpose transportation provider generally will have established its services initially through a city, county, or social service agency and most typically is established as a not-for-profit corporation. In some cases these services are operated by city or county governments; the most ambitious services are regional systems, with service areas corresponding to travel catchment areas for regional health or shopping facilities. In the 1970s some services established themselves as cooperatives, but this form of innovative organization has largely disappeared because of lack of tax advantages and available grants and loans. Most organized rural transportation systems with dispatchers and paid or volunteer vehicle drivers provide for basic nutrition and medically related trips for a specific segment of the elderly population. Discretionary trips for independent elderly residents are usually not provided, or are of low service priority (Kihl, 1990).

The typical rural transit system's operations may be controlled in several key ways. Riders may have little direct input concerning days of the week or time of day when trips are made, nor do they necessarily influence decisions concerning towns or areas served. A 1979 survey of elderly transportation found that 75% of the programs surveyed provided services other than transportation, and 83% indicated that riders had to be registered in one of these other programs before they could receive transportation services (Schauer, 1980). In addition to registration requirements, many programs have established trip priorities that further structure the travel patterns of the riders. Three-fourths of the programs in the above-cited survey said half of all their trips were regularly scheduled, and almost 90% required some sort of advance reservation. Half of the programs had no two-way radio communication with their vehicles, so routes had to be regular and changes in pickups created problems in scheduling (Schauer, 1980).

A structured approach to service delivery is primarily established out of the need to provide the most trips with the funds available. The transit manager soon discovers that a demand-responsive taxi-type service, although perhaps preferred by riders, is not a satisfactory technique for serving a large number of riders. Hence trip priorities are generally developed and a regular schedule is encouraged in an attempt to get riders to fit the available system.

It is not uncommon for rural organized transportation services to be available to the elderly only a few times a month, requiring riders to plan trips and appointments carefully. Discretionary travel to overcome isolation and to associate with one's friends and acquaintances is difficult, especially when few rural systems provide weekend service. The traditional visit to town on Saturday or a trip to church on the weekend is not possible with the typical system. The rural elderly may have their most basic life support mobility needs met, but the quality of life and feelings of well-being brought about through independence often suffer unless they can drive their own automobiles.

Financial Support of Rural Elder Mobility

Although the nonmetropolitan population contains a significantly larger proportion of economically disadvantaged people, federal expenditures per capita for human resource programs are substantially greater in metropolitan counties (Cordes, 1989). Another comparison of rural and urban area transit service funding conducted in 1990 reveals that 6% of urban systems' budgets comes from federal transit funding, whereas 31% of rural systems' budgets is from federal sources (Rucker, 1991). Although the rural areas are more dependent on federal support to maintain their rural transit systems, they receive less than 10% of the total federal transit funding available, despite the fact that 49% of the U.S. population resides in rural and small urban areas, defined as communities with less than 50,000 population (National Association for Transportation Alternatives, 1988, p. 2).

Federal support of transportation for the rural elderly derives from several sources. The U.S. Department of Transportation's Federal Transit Administration (FTA) administers funds from two sections of the Intermodal Surface Transportation Efficiency Act of 1991. Section 18 is distributed to states on a formula basis to support rural public transportation, of which a substantial portion of the ridership is elderly. Eligibility for Section 18 funding requires service to the general public, although FTA does not provide a specific measure of service that qualifies general public ridership levels (U.S. General Accounting Office, 1982). Fiscal year 1992 distributions through this program totaled $106 million. The Section 18 program has been in effect since 1978, authorized originally under the Urban Mass Transportation Act.

The Section 18 program is intended to augment rather than supplant existing transportation resources (U.S. General Accounting Office, 1982). This augmentation is an attempt to enhance economies of scale and leverage existing expenditures to increase transportation services. Larger coordinated transportation services often secure lower-cost insurance, lower-cost supplies, and other services. Section 18 has become a critical element in rural transit funding to help bring about more coordinated services.

Serving the general public and augmenting existing funds has presented a dilemma for some service providers who receive Section 18 funding. An equitable fare structure for existing social service clients and new general public riders, coupled with increased utilization of already busy equipment, has meant that the economies of scale hoped for have not always been achieved. A U.S. Department of Transportation Office of Inspector General audit of Section 18 programs in a rural state charged that grant money had been awarded to transportation providers who restrict, ignore, or discourage public transportation, and that Section 18 funds had been used by social service agencies to provide transportation services primarily for their own clientele rather than for the general public (Weaver et al., 1991).

The second FTA program of importance to transportation in rural areas is the Section 16 program. Section 16 provides capital assistance to private nonprofit agencies, tribal governments, and, in special cases, public agencies for transportation service to the elderly and persons with disabilities. Approximately $55 million was allocated on a formula basis to the states in fiscal year 1992. These funds are matched locally at a minimum level of 20%, although some states have increased local match percentage requirements to extend the state's capacity to purchase vehicles.

Other federal funding sources typically used in rural areas to support transportation for the elderly derive from programs of the U.S. Department of Health and Human Services. Although none of these programs has special set-asides for transportation, transportation is often an eligible service and allocation for this purpose is determined either at the state or local level. Title III of the Older Americans Act (OAA) is the most common non-FTA transportation source; others include the Community Services Block Grant program, Medicaid and the Social Services Block Grant program. A major complaint from service providers has been the difficulty of coordinating multiple funding sources because of variations in rules and regulations; an initiative of both FTA and the Department of Health and Human Services has been to enhance funding coordination capabilities (Bogren, 1991).

The allocation of state resources is skewed, with about 10 states accounting for nearly 90% of the nation's total state transportation funding (Rucker, 1991). In 1990, nearly 91% of this funding was targeted for urban public transportation; elderly and disabled transportation received 6% of the funding, and aid to rural public transportation constituted only 2% (Rucker, 1991).

Almost all of the rural transportation projects initiated prior to 1978 were intended to be self-supporting in some way; support was provided through fares from riders, contracts with public or private groups, and operating subsidies by some state or local governments. Although the goal of self-sufficiency is congruent with traditional rural values, a 1974 assessment of selected systems found that few had succeeded in becoming self-supporting (U.S. Senate, Committee on Agriculture and Forestry, 1974). Most rural passenger systems request some fare or contribution, but farebox cost recovery has been problematic because of low demand and the inability of rural elders to pay fares sufficient to support the service. The Older Americans Act prohibits charging even a small fare, further complicating systems' ability to recover a share of operational costs. Even though fares are prohibited on OAA-supported systems, elders have indicated that paying one dollar for a trip, or more for longer-distance rural trips, is fair for those who can afford it (National Eldercare Institute on Transportation, 1992b).

Given the typical lack of financial self-sufficiency by systems serving the rural elderly and the escalating competition for federal funds, agencies raise funds in ways that make budgeting difficult. Generating local match through bake sales, fish fries, and quilt raffles is common for rural transit systems. The services often operate with modestly paid staff and are financially tenuous.

Challenges and Responses for Sustaining Rural Transportation Services

Beyond the challenge of financing rural transportation services, a number of planning- and service-related considerations affect the ability to provide quality service to rural elders. Tools with which to make appropriate decisions about service design, consistent or relevant standards to apply to rural service, and human resource development represent three specific challenges. Sustaining rural transportation services requires systematic approaches to the special development needs of rural provider agencies.

Appropriate Planning Methods and Tools

In 1977, Tardiff, Lam, and Dana observed that "the state of the art in nonmetropolitan transportation planning is one in which there has been considerable disjointed effort in providing services, but little systematic development in policies, planning theories and methods" (p. 33). Little progress has been made since that statement was made. In a 1991 review of transportation services for the elderly, the U.S. General Accounting Office found that 10 of 19 studies reviewed "cited inadequate data as a barrier to maximizing the benefits of special transportation funding" (p. 11). Systematic research for estimating demand and predicting ridership through the use of statistical models has not been conducted, nor are there national data on the service characteristics of special transportation services.

The definition of unmet need and the policies for providing service have progressed little since 1977. However, many rural systems have been designed and planned following a standard planning process modeled after urban systems, where objectives are stated, an implementation plan is developed, and services are delivered. The assumption that programs designed for urban settings can be transplanted to meet rural needs ignores issues unique to rural communities.

The Federal Transit Administration has never published rural and small urban transportation planning requirements. The Administration on Aging requires a service planning program, and some states have adopted requirements for three- or five-year plans. For example, since 1979 the state of North Carolina has recommended the 20-step planning process outlined in Table 3.1.

Despite the fact that rigorous planning methods and tools are not available, a planning process with a strong component of community involvement should be followed (Miller & Goodnight, 1973). Particular emphasis on public involvement in rural planning is important, because no matter how sophisticated and detailed, common analytic techniques do not provide completely accurate estimates of transit patronage in smaller communities. Community input combined with testing the most promising alternatives is the most feasible approach, because the cost of error is not as great as in larger systems. Changes in routes or service level can be tested at little additional cost.

Factors entering into the decisions pertinent to implementation include social, political, economic, and technical considerations. The

Table 3.1 Twenty Planning Steps

---

1. Form steering committee.

2. Hold preliminary meeting.[a]

3. Gather background information on county.

4. Inventory public bus operator.

5. Inventory taxi and private bus operators.

6. Inventory human service agencies.

7. Summarize existing arrangements among providers.

8. Present inventory data to steering committee.[a]

9. Identify and enumerate user groups.

10. Identify public transportation trip needs of user groups.

11. Identify trip needs of human service agencies.

12. Identify unmet needs.

13. Identify major attractors and generators.

14. Present trip needs, unmet demands to steering committee.[a]

15. Revise goals, discuss objectives.[a]

16. List and analyze alternatives.[a]

17. Choose service design.[a]

18. Detail the chosen service design.

19. Adopt procedures for updating and evaluation.[a]

20. Get county commissioner adoption.

SOURCE: Adapted from North Carolina Department of Transportation (1979, p. 4).
a. Step requires meeting of the steering committee.

transportation-related estimate should be balanced in accordance to the role each of these considerations plays. Areas of consideration range from service design and farebox recovery to accessibility features of the service to meet requirements of the Americans with Disabilities Act (Table 3.2).

Among the most difficult areas to assess are cost, service evaluation, and pricing. Pricing policy is critical in light of the dismal financial record of many systems. Policies should carefully weigh the choice

Table 3.2 Governing Body Policy Decision Areas

Farebox recovery

Special fares

Geographic area of service (demand responsive)

Designation of priority patron (demand responsive)

Designation of priority trip purpose (demand responsive)

Client eligibility requirements (if applicable)

Client billing rates, form, and amount (if applicable)

Fleet deployment and garaging

Vehicle maintenance scheduling

Capital replacement

Hours of service

Length and location of routes (fixed route)

Days of service

Level of service (for example, fixed-route headways)

Vehicle capacity and vehicle type

Ultimate fleet size

Vehicle backup

Accessibility features

SOURCE: Adapted from National Association of County Engineers (1986, p. 3-2).

between fares and suggested donations, based on several considerations: avoiding the stigma attached to free fare systems as "welfare buses," generating revenue to minimize subsidies, allocating scarce resources among potential users, and attaching costs to the benefits perceived by the users (Tardiff et al., 1977).

Service Delivery Standards

A critical issue for rural elderly transit service is the development of a rational service delivery mechanism and service level expectation. A desired minimum level of service for individuals has been difficult to establish, and no standard level of service exists that can be compared with other rural services. Public standards developed for services such as rural postal delivery, elementary and secondary education, and farm-to-market roads are reasonably understood by the public and used to judge performance. For example, postal service is offered six days a week as a minimum standard, a standard that is understood and accepted by the public. In education, although there are criticisms of lack of sufficient quality, rural youth are expected to attend school through four years of high school to attain a diploma. Farm-to-market roads are maintained at least at a minimum to support the economic base of rural areas.

No comparable service standards have been developed for rural elderly transportation that then are translated into cost estimates that would allow a funding scheme to develop as has occurred for postal service, education, and farm-to-market roads. With the development of service standards, the question of who will pay could then be addressed, and a reasonable balance of funding support could be found among the user and all levels of government: local, state, and federal. In the absence of widely held service standards and agreed-upon measurements, the general evaluation theory, which is most useful when compared with other evaluation techniques, is the cost-effectiveness measure to assess the relative value of any expenditure.

Lee, Tamakloe, and Mulinazzi (1981) found that the cost-effectiveness measure is preferable to other evaluation techniques, such as cost-benefit ratios, goal achievement or impact incidents, and matrix rating and ranking methods. However, it is helpful to utilize the goal achievement method as a precursor to the cost-effectiveness measure. The goal achievement method looks at the achievement of the essential goals of the service, such as increasing access to nutrition or health care facilities or some other broad goal, and then places a cost-effectiveness measure on the outcome of the services meeting that goal. Cost-effectiveness is always subject to definition in the particular area where the service is being provided. The diversity of services and operating environments in rural areas has created challenges to those who attempt comparisons among rural systems. As an alternative to comparisons among systems, the planning process for local systems should include establishing target costs for the service and then determining if the costs per trip, per vehicle mile, or per some other measure are reasonable for the operating environment.

Again, the difficulty of comparing rural areas is illustrated by the federal processes established through FTA, which has a prescribed planning process and conducts a triennial review of its urban projects. In rural areas, no such review exists. Fiscal audits typically are conducted, but program audits and performance reviews usually are not conducted. Program audits and reviews are important to a thorough and systematic planning process if system performance is to be enhanced.

Trained Human Resource Pool: Drivers to Board Members

The lack of a trained labor pool has inhibited rural transportation services on at least three levels. First, leadership on boards of directors and project advisory committees may be poorly trained and inexperienced with regard to operating a community service or business. The advisory boards, although well intentioned with respect to meeting the needs of the elderly, may be poorly versed in the operations of a social service. Second, the manager and staff of the service itself may be poorly trained and inexperienced. It is common for managers of rural services to come up through the ranks, well versed in the operations and provision of service but possessing inadequate program planning and administration skills. Finally, the community support and available labor for mechanical, financial, legal, computer management, and other technical support may simply be unavailable in rural areas or poorly trained in transportation agency needs. For example, local maintenance shops may be ill equipped to repair bus air conditioners and hydraulic lift equipment typically operated by a rural transit system, requiring transport of vehicles in need of repair to distant communities, incurring long delays in service and significant costs.

Indeed, the staff may require substantial direction and encouragement, as wages are typically low and needed skills involve getting things done in a hands-on fashion rather than systematic management of data and achievement of goals, objectives, and targets. There is no college or preparatory degree program offered in rural transit management. Although recent national and state initiatives to improve access to rural transit training and technical assistance have grown with the aid of federal funds, the relative isolation of these systems often leads to their reinventing solutions that neighboring projects or other services have already perfected. Typical rural managers, particularly those in very small agencies, are not well read in the field of management or transportation literature, and may not be active in their state transit associations.

At least three efforts are required to overcome the lack of management expertise in rural areas. First, periodic management reviews should be conducted to note deficiencies in management of services, noting areas for remedial learning and outlining a course of action for managers' self-help, including a basic list of readings. Second, managers should be encouraged to take "busman's holidays." By visiting one or more similar-sized transit services each year, managers would be exposed to other operations' solutions to service problems. Third, the most ambitious effort is the development of a course of study for managers of rural elderly transit programs. This course of study would be similar to an associate degree offered by a community college and would allow a manager to secure a certificate of training over a period of time representing formal course work, readings, and investigation directed at issues of rural elderly transit.

Labor pool issues for support services such as maintenance are more difficult, because those may be contracted services. The lack of service workers who are knowledgeable about wheelchair lifts and associated hydraulic and bus mechanics is a particular problem in rural areas. Buses have many similarities to large trucks or modified vans, but some peculiarities do exist. As a result, the vehicles tend to be undermaintained, warranty work is inconvenient, and securing settlement for warranty work is often difficult. When a vehicle has to be towed a hundred miles or trailered a long distance, disagreements concerning who pays for a replacement vehicle or who pays for the transportation for warranty work are troublesome. Furthermore, identifying maintenance suppliers who employ environmentally sound practices, such as recycling air-conditioning freon and properly disposing of petroleum products and antifreeze, are issues to which managers should be alert. Managers who seek qualified mechanics who employ environmentally sound practices are even more limited in their options.

The need for manager training is clear when one reviews specific program operations. In a review of volunteer programs in Minnesota, it was discovered that only 48% of the responding programs checked volunteer drivers for valid driver's licenses, and that only 43% of the programs checked for proof of insurance (Independent Transportation Management Services, 1990). These basic management issues are elements that an alert board and manager should include as standard operating procedure. Evidence of such omissions supports the argument that there is a need for simplified training manuals and courses of instruction. Simplified accounting manuals and operations procedures manuals for the various types of services need to be developed. Training is essential to improve the understanding of the elements of a quality management program.

Active and involved boards improve a community's sense of worth and ability to maintain and take care of its citizens. However, the complexity of transit service requires board members who are savvy and can provide adequate direction for staff. Honorary board positions are no longer sufficient. Boards need transit governance training, with periodic updates—at least yearly—on topics of current importance. Only specific training in transportation and management can provide board members with the leadership skills required today.

Research and Policy Issues: Implications for Practitioners

The last comprehensive examination of transportation services and older people was conducted by the Department of Health and Human Resources in 1980, sponsored by the U.S. Administration on Aging. Since 1980, little systematic research has been conducted on rural elderly transportation. The FTA has published descriptive and technical reports on a regular basis about topics of related interest to rural elderly transportation providers, but federal research money for transit declined to rather critical levels during the 1980s (Smerk, 1991). Basic research on the value of transit service to a community in economic and social terms is unavailable. Krout (1986) notes that some basic research about rural elderly transportation is not available and questions how the rural elderly are affected by the lack of transportation and the costs and benefits (economical, physical, and psychological) of these transportation patterns. When transportation problems exist for rural elderly, how can they be most effectively and appropriately overcome? Systematic inquiries into desirable minimum levels of service, demand, and use of service do not exist in current literature.

Research Needs

Despite the lack of research about transportation services for the rural elderly, there is no question that older people need transportation. Questions posed in the 1980 report *Improving Transportation Services for Older Americans* are valid today, despite being more than 10 years old (Institute of Public Administration, 1980). How much transportation should be provided? What kind of service should be provided and who should supply it? In the face of rising prices and costs, energy shortages, and limited budgets, how should we pay for it? These basic research questions have not been approached systematically, although surveys regularly show transportation as one of the elderly's greatest needs. In a two-year national study of rural Area Agencies on Aging, transportation was the most frequently mentioned service need (Krout, 1989a). In a Texas Department of Aging needs assessment conducted in 1990, transportation was cited as the greatest need of the elderly (Sharp, 1991).

So many surveys have regularly cited transportation as a problem that a certain frustration is recognizable in the aging network. This frustration focuses on the fact that considerable sums of money are spent on transportation each year (the Administration on Aging estimated that $68 million from Title III of the Older Americans Act was spent for transportation in fiscal year 1989), yet transportation still is regularly mentioned as a high need area (U.S. General Accounting Office, 1991). The questions remain: How much transportation should be provided? What kind? Who should pay for it and how?

Policy Issues

Rural Transportation as a Legitimate Service

The recognition of rural transportation as a legitimate service component has been rapid and wholehearted from the standpoint of social service providers. Service providers in the 1960s recognized that without transportation, very often the services they were offering could not be used. However, those outside the social services network often do not recognize the need for special services for the elderly because they themselves have automobiles and may not know anyone who is dependent on others for their mobility requirements. In practically every community there are several transportation services, and Americans have shown a willingness to support a highly specialized, fragmented transit service for specific identified needs, such as for Head Start programs, for sheltered workshops for the developmentally disabled, and, most notably, for schoolchildren in general. It is possible that Americans will not broadly support general public rural transportation but will support transportation for the elderly, the disabled, and children. However, the fact that future generations will expect higher levels of mobility than do current generations is not widely recognized. U.S. society today is highly mobile, and as current generations age, more comprehensive general public services for the rural elderly will need to be developed, so use of fragmented services such as school buses becomes more important.

Opportunities exist for joint use of school buses, although few states have implemented such programs. Agencies involved with services for the elderly should work with the school systems to share use of school buses, particularly for transportation to nutrition sites at midday, when most school fleets are partially idle. By allowing the elderly to use school buses, school boards could have an opportunity to secure elderly support for schools and school bond issues.

Who Will Pay? Distributing Service Costs in Society

Americans have enjoyed a subsidized highway and automobile system for many years. The cost of gasoline does not fully cover the environmental or social costs of the automobile, and the private sector notions of profit for transit services and full cost recovery often implied in evaluation measures are not entirely equitable. It is unlikely that a cost-benefit ratio could be developed successfully now for the interstate highway system, and yet transit services are routinely required to develop such measures.

The cost of maintaining people in their own homes is lower than that for maintaining them in institutionalized settings, and provision of transportation services is often a critical element in people's ability to remain in their own homes. The aging network should be alert to the costs incurred when individuals are not able to stay in their homes because of a lack of transportation, and to the long-run savings of providing such individuals with transportation services.

Public-Private Cooperation

As is the trend in government services, more public-private cooperative efforts are being initiated to solve the complex problems of our society. The bellwether approach taken for the 1984 Olympics, when corporate sponsorship helped generate the first profitable Olympic

Games, is being repeated in a variety of efforts, from garbage collection to provision of mass transportation. Allowing the market and individuals to provide for mobility requirements is often highly successful, particularly in urban areas, but in rural areas the lack of available entrepreneurs and existing providers has lessened the opportunity for private sector participation. The aging network should be alert to any local transportation providers, such as taxi, charter bus, or school bus operators, who may have the qualifications necessary to provide passenger transportation in a rural setting, and should encourage them by offering contracts and incentives.

Coordinating With All Transportation Modes

The lack of coordination among rural transportation modes characteristic of rural planning and operations translates to fewer travel options for rural elders (U.S. Department of Agriculture, 1991). Little coordination exists between private social service transportation, rural public transportation, intercity buses or trains, and airlines. Even less exists between passenger transportation systems and infrastructure planning to consider alternative designs.

Federal efforts to improve coordination between Department of Transportation-funded services and Department of Health and Human Services-funded programs, state initiatives such as those in Florida and Kansas to mandate transportation coordination, some local initiatives aimed at coordination, and public-private coordination programs such as the Rural Connector Program sponsored by Greyhound Lines, Inc., illustrate a move in the direction of improved network coordination. Further, the Intermodal Surface Transportation Efficiency Act of 1991 includes new intermodal planning requirements; local governments and states must consider modal interaction of planning decisions and transferability of some funds between highways and transit. This may at least improve the dialogue between the two sectors.

Land-Use Policy Considerations in Rural Transportation Design

Even in rural settings, the polycentric mode of development is apparent. An older central business district may be eclipsed on the outskirts of town by a shopping center development requiring motorized transportation for access. Most small rural communities in the past could be easily accessed by walking, but with developments now being made outside city cores, walking is not an option. Ideally, before plans for senior centers, clinics, or other human services are developed, passenger transportation should be considered. How are the rural elderly going to get there? The range of options, from walking to driving to use of transit services, should be analyzed and used appropriately.

Walking will increase in importance in any community where social services exist, providing the pedestrian network is satisfactory. Indeed, it can be shown that a community must be "pedestrian friendly" before it can be "transit friendly." This means it must be easy to walk from one's residence to the street or other point at which one meets a transportation vehicle, whether it is a private automobile or a public transit vehicle. Amenities such as benches, canopies, and well-marked paths through parking lots and other developments are necessary to enhance the opportunities for walking. Even parking lots at senior centers should be considered and improved, as they are a common battlefield for nicks and dents in the private automobile and difficult for pedestrians. Walking across some senior center parking lots that have no well-marked pedestrian paths or crosswalks is dangerous. New parking lots in future developments should allow extra space for parked vehicles and improved walkways for pedestrians.

Government Regulatory and Funding Policies

Little doubt exists that the role of government will increase, particularly in regard to the environmental regulations of passenger transportation. Clean Air Act requirements and Clean Water Act requirements with respect to runoff from parking lots and seepage from underground tanks are highly regulated and likely to continue. National environmental policies should recognize the positive relationship between transit and environmental health of this country through reduced reliance on single-occupant transportation, yet hold the transit industry accountable for responsible behavior through compliance with emissions standards through equipment maintenance, utilization of appropriate alternative fuels technology, recycling, and planning and maintenance of its physical plant.

Summary and Conclusions

The environment for rural elderly transportation is a complex one; few planning or research tools are available, and practitioners must provide services with staffs and boards that are not well versed in the operations of passenger transportation. The emphasis should be on training boards and staff members, to enhance their capabilities in management and evaluation of services. Boards should be progressive and alert to the transportation needs of social services being developed and to land-use patterns. Transportation advisory boards should insist that passenger transportation needs be considered concurrent with the development of social services or land-use plans.

Issues of equity with regard to government expenditures in rural areas should be pursued by the aging network. Further, the ability of individuals to contribute to or pay for services should be evaluated, and the possibility of using a sliding scale or means test for individuals to pay for services should be investigated.

Research on transportation services for the rural elderly is needed, particularly regarding evaluation measures, planning tools, and the establishment of criteria that will place transportation as a component of any rural community. For elder transportation to become a component of the rural community, criteria for levels of service must be established and the community must be educated about the needs of the elderly and the adoption of those criteria.

4

Case Management
in a Rural Setting

ENE KRISTI URV-WONG
DONNA McDOWELL

An Overview of the Nature of
and Need for Case Management

Originated as a means of coordinating services to individuals with complex needs, the case management process has evolved into a sociopolitical beast with great momentum, but uncertain direction. Viewed as a panacea for the rampant fragmentation of long-term care services in the 1980s, bits and pieces, but seldom the whole, of the case management process were quickly adopted by both rural and urban agencies and organizations. Disagreement over the definition of the term *case management* and the lack of a universal model of case management resulted in practices that assumed much and in programs of varying shapes, sizes, and effectiveness.

The Need for Case Management in Rural Areas

The greatest need for case management arises for people who have complex and multiple physical, psychological, and social needs. Such frail individuals live everywhere, but those who live in rural areas often find their problems exacerbated by the characteristics of rural economics and demographic characteristics, such as distances between those with needs and service providers; the availability of services, for example, respite or mental health services; the out-migration of younger people from rural areas, resulting in a small hiring pool of professionals or paraprofessionals and a loosening of traditional family ties (i.e., traditional family caregivers); and the lack of a firm economic basis for attracting new services or individuals to the area.

Goals of Case Management

The commonly accepted goals of case management are as follows: assessment of the needs of an individual; obtainment of appropriate-quality services to ameliorate the needs of that individual; and program cost containment, that is, using resources in the most cost-effective manner. Case management is resource management (Austin, 1983). The process draws from a finite pool of energy, time, and money.

In addition to explicitly stated goals, underlying goals may coexist with program goals; such underlying goals may include serving in a gatekeeping function to determine who receives services, creating a single point of contact for clients in need of immediate care, and tracking both client outcome and the performance of service providers (Kane, 1988). When explicit and unspoken goals coexist, dangerous assumptions may arise that can lead to inappropriate use of services, and thereby a waste of scarce resources.

Models of Case Management

Models of case management that operate in rural and urban settings are based on resource constraints. For example, the broker model, service management model, and managed care model (Austin, 1988), and, similarly, the five models described by Kane, Penrod, Davidson, Moscovice, and Rich (1989), are based on economic incentives that are potentially counterproductive to serving the best interest of clients.

The Makeup of Case Management: Driving Variables

Although case management programs can be classified by their reimbursement or payment mechanisms, there are additional flexible variables that drive the makeup of a program and allow it to "fit" its environment. Such variables include the program's purpose or mission, its primary program function, its targeting strategy, its staffing levels and credentialing, its optimal caseload, and its expected duration for the delivery of services. The purpose or mission of a particular program, such as limiting or minimizing the use of nursing homes, is a chief variable in determining the makeup of that program. The mission is the yardstick against which all of the actions of a program are measured to determine if the programs is on track. Funding sources may predetermine the mission of a program as well its function: that of advocate, working on behalf of clients to obtain service dollars or services, or that of gatekeeper, assuring that only those individuals in specific need of services obtain services. The function or role that a case management program assumes—whether advocate, gatekeeper, or a hybrid—also regulates how clients respond to an individual case manager or program (Urv-Wong, 1990). Programs that lack any formal guidelines invite individuals working in the system to develop and adopt their own rationale. For example, program planners or fieldworkers may confuse the purpose of a program and its function, deciding independently, for instance, that the reason a program exists is to keep accurate records for funding agencies (Urv-Wong & Kane, 1989).

The target population, the defined service population of a case management program, also defines the parameters of the program. The complex and special needs of a specific population—for example, the developmentally disabled, the frail elderly, or persons with AIDS—determine the types of services utilized and the distinct knowledge base needed by case managers in order to be effective. If, however, no clear definition of a target population exists, case managers may err when determining who should be served. That is, they may conclude that everyone should receive case management (neither cost-efficient nor true), or they may err on the side of overexuberant gatekeeping, and set strict eligibility guidelines for program access (inadvertently denying access to those in true need). Whereas a potential client may decline services because of his or her innately independent nature, because he or she disagrees with prescribed case plans, or because of family interference, but declining services do not diminish the existence of need. Nor should it jeopardize the client's right to future or alternative services.

A major problem of targeting a particular population for service is that of confusing the family of the client with the client. Although client families can play a key role in care planning or as informal care providers, pressure from family members is often counterproductive to resolution of client-based problems and dilemmas. Programs that operate in rural environments are especially vulnerable to family pressures because of the nature of the small, tight-knit community structure.

Another compelling variable contributing to the makeup of a program is that of staffing; issues involved include the levels of staffing necessary to conduct an effective program and credential standards for staff. Programs that base qualifications of case managers solely on minimum education standards ignore the importance of specialized knowledge of a targeted client base, as well as familiarity with local services. This consideration is especially important in rural areas, which, because of geographic isolation and funding constraints, often depend on local labor pools to staff programs.

Caseload limitations may also be set by funding agencies, but more often caseload is determined by the number of case managers an agency can afford and the number of clients it is allowed or can afford to serve. Lacking guidelines, a vital question becomes, What is an optimal caseload? Two factors can determine optimal caseload for a program: the definition of *case management* to which an agency adheres and the makeup of the target population, which, in turn, drives intensity of service (Urv-Wong, 1990). When determining optimal caseload, rural program planners should include additional time factors for travel, assessment, and monitoring. The best way to determine optimal caseload is to monitor individual care plans to determine whether or not they are being adequately fulfilled.

Service provision should not be viewed as indefinite. Case management programmers and policy makers must set time parameters for all services. Psychologically, approaching a client in terms of indefinite services, as opposed to assuming an established reassessment timetable, can blind a case manager to actual improvement in a client's condition. Furthermore, indefinite service provision may prove a disservice to clients who become overdependent.

How It Works

Case management has been compared to a Rorschach test (Kane, 1990), described as "telling us more about the particular case manager than about case management." That is, how case management is practiced is a function of how individuals interpret whatever parameters or guidelines (however minimal) are issued to them.

Elements of Case Management

Functional areas that should be present in a program in order to define it as case management include case finding or outreach, intake, multi-dimensional assessment, care planning, service acquisition, monitoring (of care plan and services), and reassessment/case closure.

Case Finding

Case finding is designed to locate individuals who might benefit from services. An important distinction in outreach is that not everyone needs case management; furthermore, not everyone who needs it, wants it.

Outreach is essential in rural areas, where funds can be severely limited. Rural areas must rely on word-of-mouth and one-to-one contacts; churches and other religious organizations, fraternal groups, and service organizations may function as community focal points for outreach efforts.

Intake/Screening

The intake process includes obtaining basic information about a client. The actual depth of information obtained varies with the need or desire to differentiate clients in a program. Screening allows quick identification of indicators of the probable complexity of needs of a particular client. Intake is the process of identifying the target population by applying abbreviated, cost-effective, yet reasonable objective indicators of need, such as presenting problem, age, income, living arrangement, current level of both formal and informal services, or level of disability (deficiencies in activities of daily living [ADLs] and instrumental activities of daily living [IADLs]). The cost-benefit of screening should be seen as a primary component of the intake function.

Often in rural areas intake consists of nothing more than recording a name, a phone number, and perhaps a presenting problem. These referrals are passed on to a case manager, who must determine from either minimal information or additional contacts whether case management services are appropriate. At the polar opposite, some rural agencies confuse intake screening with multidimensional assessment and conduct a full assessment on every individual who calls. The rationale given by case management administrators in these agencies is that the assessments are completed "just in case" the individuals need services (Urv-Wong, 1990).

Multidimensional Assessment

The baseline multidimensional assessment gathers crucial information for the case management process. Such a tool allows for easy transfer of information among agencies. It also avoids duplication of effort—that is, the completion of multiple assessments—which not only exhausts case management resources but may also exhaust and confuse the client, because assessment instruments vary in scope and in depth, from a few simple questions to intensive 30-page documents. The level of trust developed between assessor and client during the assessment is key to the quality of information obtained.

A recent study of case management in rural areas determined the following to be the most common areas assessed: physical well-being and medical history (99% of the sample), psychological or mental functioning (97%), functional ability (that is, ADL/IADL; 96%), social inventories (96%), survey of formal (88%) and informal services (94%), economic and financial position (89%), in-home safety surveys (93%), and family relationships (92%) (Krout, 1991a). Additionally, either assessments should include implicit questions or case managers should receive training in eliciting clients' goals and preferences for care.

A fierce argument ensues in case management practice regarding the need for comprehensive assessment when relatively few services are available, as in many rural areas. Why, for example, should a case manager assess a client's psychological needs when no counseling services exist within a 50-mile radius? The counterargument is that conducting an assessment, regardless of the availability of any particular services, provides a case manager with a baseline measurement from which to track an individual's progress or decline. In addition, when formal services do become available, the need is already documented. The assessment provides a record of risk factors that should be monitored, even if services are not available and no service plan exists.

Care Planning

Care planning is a vital process. It is not, however, a single static finding or document (although a written care plan is a result of the process). "It is through the care plan that the system is made operational" (Schneider, 1988). The care plan is a vital link for clear and concise communication between the client and the case manager and between service providers and the case manager. Furthermore, obtaining client input and approval of the care plan can enhance client understanding and compliance.

Care planning translates the root problems discovered during the multidimensional assessment into need statements. Need statements are used in conjunction with a client's values and preferences to set desired outcome goals and to design a care plan of informal and formal services that best meets the needs of the individual.

Rural case managers may suggest that, given their intimate knowledge of their clients, storing information "in their heads" is less time-consuming than preparing written care plans and is therefore more efficient. Given the amount of detail inherent to a good care plan, however, how fair or efficient is it if a case manager "forgets" some fact, or fails to note a change in a patient's condition?

Care plans should not be confused with service plans. In rural areas many individuals complete service plans and call them care plans. Care plans must describe the type of problem the client has and the planned outcomes of the services. Care planning must be "problem oriented and goal directed" (Schneider, 1988).

Service Acquisition

Care planning and service acquisition are interrelated. Case managers often function as client advocates, obtaining the services that clients and their families need, and as service gatekeepers, assuring that only those who really require and can potentially benefit from services receive them. How a case management program handles service acquisition depends on which economic model it most resembles. For example, in a broker model, case managers have no actual service dollars to spend on clients, but are still responsible for client referral and follow-up (Austin, 1988; Kane et al., 1989).

Monitoring

Monitoring is a vital quality assurance function of case managers. It should include, but not be limited to, monitoring client satisfaction with the plan, the service element of case management (quality, timeliness, duration), and the care planning element (appropriateness of the care plan). Care plan monitoring is the constant reevaluation or fine tuning of the care plan in order to assure that the original goals of the plan are met.

Reassessment

An assessment is only a snapshot in time. Typically clients experience improvements and declines of chronic conditions and social support systems. Periodic review is necessary to establish the viability of the baseline assessment and care plan over time. Good practice dictates setting a schedule of reassessment per an established timetable or on a preestablished case-by-case basis. Such a timetable is a minimum standard, not a maximum. In some rural areas monitoring may become very informal, and this can be dangerous. Without a uniform and formal monitoring system, the probability of clients "falling through the cracks" is high.

Standard and Alternative Systems

Rural Approaches and Options

Case management in rural areas can take many forms. These forms are often dictated by historical precedent, such as the design of existing programs. Other variables include responses to sociopolitical forces in a community and the perception and interpretation of administrative necessity (Urv-Wong, 1990). Three general rationales for providing case management in rural areas are coordination, priority setting, and record keeping (Urv-Wong, 1990). Although, to an extent, each of these rationales is vital, and none can stand alone.

Coordination

Coordination is the strongest rationale provided by rural agencies for providing case management services, but it is valid only if it includes the completed bundle of services from outreach to reassessment. Most important, even if all the components of case management exist, unless they are coordinated and integrated into a system, they do not necessarily constitute case management. Many small rural agencies claim to provide case management services when they merely coordinate transportation and nutrition services (Urv-Wong, 1990). Staff shortages may lead agencies to employ "transportation case managers" or even "nutrition case managers." This results in a service-based model of case management. Such a model results in many case managers, but little case management (see Figure 4.1) (Urv-Wong, 1990).

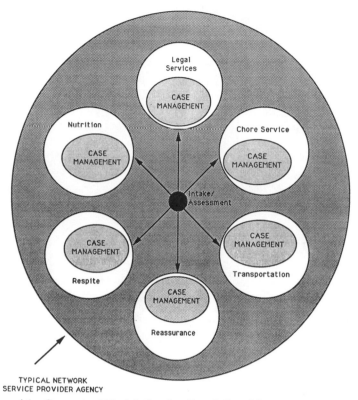

Figure 4.1. Conceptual Model: Service-Based Case Management
SOURCE: Urv-Wong (1990).

In a service-based model a single assessment may be conducted and passed to each service-based case manager, or each individual service center may conduct its own assessment and keep its own files on each client. Information flows between each service-based case manager and the client, but not among the various service-based case managers. The weakness of the system emanates from operating multiple contact points, with little communication and many opportunities to develop service gaps. Often in rural areas this model occurs because of staff shortages or simply because particular service centers are pervasive in the system. To change a service-based model, individuals in each service center need to look beyond themselves to the agency level of operation and then place the agency within the context of the overall continuum of

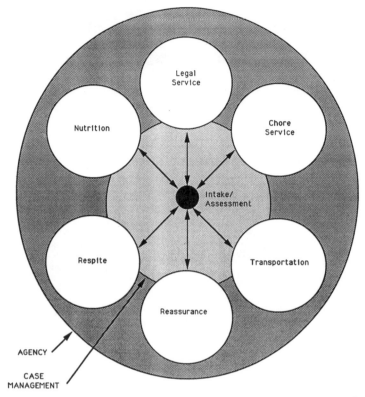

Figure 4.2. Conceptual Model: Case Management as an Overlay to Existing Structure
SOURCE: Urv-Wong (1990).

long-term care. Each service center must trust and use a single assessment and coordinate care planning through staff care planning conferences.

In contrast, Figure 4.2 illustrates what might be referred to as a classic model of case management (Urv-Wong, 1990). This figure shows the case manager as the primary contact between the various service centers and the client. It adheres to the rule, "Thou shalt have only one case manager" (Kane, 1990).

The great conceptual strength of case management is its ability to "function as an overlay to existing organizational structure with minimal disruption to existing practice" (Austin, 1983), therefore, the key is to use the existing superstructure of an agency, rather than reinvent the wheel. This usually involves enhancing communication among all parts of the agency. The small informal structure of rural agencies sometimes tends toward informal management and monitoring. Informality should not, however, be confused with flexibility. Although a formalized system has parameters and guidelines, it should have enough flexibility to allow it to work with clients from particular geographic or sociopolitical circumstances.

Priority Setting

Priority setting is a model of overexuberant gatekeeping. Such a model strictly controls who will receive services through the use of a hierarchical ranking of client need (Urv-Wong, 1990). Those with the highest score receive services. If someone with greater need appears, individuals may be "bumped" from services. It operates when agencies or organizations fail to receive targeting information, make assumptions, and proceed on their own. Priority setting is dangerous. It removes professional judgment from the case management process.

Record Keeping

Record keeping is a necessary and vital component of case management. Not only must client records be kept, but also administrative records regarding costs and contracts, and any other files required by funding agencies. The problems occur when keeping accurate and up-to-date records becomes all-pervasive, when record keeping becomes more important than the client.

Although it is true that some funding agencies require a plethora of forms and files in order to maintain funding levels, if similar incentives to provide quality and appropriate care are lacking, such agencies should not be surprised when case management programs do a better job at maintaining files than they do at serving clients. Counterproductive incentives must be recognized by an agency and balanced with its mission.

In a Rural Agency

The Rural Difference

The major issues facing case management in rural areas include resource restraints and geography. Not only are many case managers working only part-time, many also fulfill more than one role. In such situations, case managers and their supervisors need real consistency about which clients should receive case management, and should establish solid methods and procedures for record keeping and client tracking. Client preferences may need to be balanced with the availability of services (especially transportation).

In some rural agencies, program planners describe what they believe are differing levels of case management. For example, some see information and referral (I&R) as the first level. Although I&R is a component of case management, it alone does not constitute a case management program, or even a level of case management. It is a key element of community services, but it is only I&R, nothing more. Furthermore, individuals who require only I&R services do not require the intensive attention of case management services.

Apparently, everyone wants to be a case manager and to offer case management. Many agency programs are organized around two or three services; although these may be essential to a good community services program, unless they deliver a full package of coordinated case management functions, they cannot be classified as case management programs. Such agencies may provide very necessary services to their communities, services their clients would find it difficult to function without, but they are not practicing case management. The key is for all agencies to accept their functions for what they are, do the best possible job, and not burden themselves with self-important labels that do not apply.

In rural areas with limited formal service resources, case managers need an abundance of flexibility, inspiration, and authority to "create" services from existing community resources. This includes using unconventional service locations and providers, gaining access to funds for equipment and home modifications that may reduce the need for direct services, and allowing competent individuals to take some risks. Rural case managers may have real advantages over their urban counterparts because of their knowledge of local people who may be willing to "help out" in voluntary ways to supplement purchased services.

Strengths of Rural Case Management

In addition, rural agencies have specific strengths to capitalize upon (Urv-Wong, 1990). Small agencies can avoid the red tape of bigger bureaucracies and often have loyal staffs who understand and are committed to an area and its people. In addition, the informal communications networks (i.e., the grapevines) of small communities, although inappropriate for use in client services monitoring, are excellent means for tackling common problems of interagency coordination and quick response to emergencies.

Issues in Developing and Providing Case Management

Particular issues are common to almost all case management programs, such as conflicting definitions, lack of adequate services, questions of targeting, controlling funding and administrative costs, and staff credentialing. Although these concerns are present regardless of location, programs in rural areas may experience such problems to a greater degree than those in urban areas.

Definitions

Discrepancies in definitions occur between official documentation and practitioner perceptions of case management, among professionals in the field, and between organizations practicing case management and agencies reimbursing for the service. These discrepancies can lead to major battles over jurisdiction, territory, and clients. These turf battles occur primarily because of the lack of an acceptable definition for the expected goals of case management.

Perhaps the fundamental or baseline definition of case management is provided by Rosalie Kane (1988): "Case management is the coordination of a specific group of resources and services for a specific group of people." Further, Monika White (1987) defines case management as "a service function directed at coordinating existing resources to assure appropriate and continuous care for individuals on a case by case basis." Although terminology varies, the basic theory must remain constant.

Administrative Costs

The case management process adds certain administrative costs to a program. These include increased time on documentation and time spent monitoring specific cases. Although additional record keeping is necessary, the time spent is an active investment rather than a burden or barrier to care. The cost-benefit of case management must be weighed against the cost of additional labor. An often-heard criticism of additional paperwork is that such documentation acts as a barrier. Case managers often believe that the more time they spend with clients, the better their ability to serve those clients. However, quality is more a function of how time is spent rather than how much time is spent with a client.

Lack of Services/Restriction of Services

Lack of services in a specific area can be viewed as a lack or shortage of formal service organizations, as limited access to formal agencies, or as limited availability of informal services provided by family or friends. Although a key component of case management, formal community services should never supplant informal services. Instead, they should complement and support the informal service structure.

Although formal service options may be limited or even restricted by funding sources, informal services are limited only by a case manager's imagination. Too often, case management programs limit available service options for individuals because they lack a history with a specific service provider; because a supervisor discourages innovative use of an existing service because it has never been tried; because case managers limit their service acquisition to services provided by their own agencies (a clear conflict of interest) or because funding agency guidelines restrict efficacious or creative use of available funding; or because it is simply easier to produce "cookie-cutter" care plans. Such counterproductive actions can close the door to available, preferred, and perhaps even cost-saving options for the client and the program.

Although all necessary services will never exist in some rural areas, one thing always will: waiting lists. A common debate in many case management programs is whether to keep waiting lists, especially long lists. Placing a potential client on a waiting list, particularly if he or she has a low priority, is viewed as making a tacit promise of services, a promise that many case managers feel can never be fulfilled. This conflict contrasts with the administrative need to keep waiting lists current in order to illustrate the growing need for service.

Funding

Money, and its particular source, is one of the primary determinants of program structure. Although many programs predetermine who may be served by issuing strict guidelines, many others do not provide specific guidance. Therefore, case managers are often assigned the task of determining who is most in need. This is an unfair burden to place on fieldworkers. It can be hoped that their work translates in such cases to "those who would most benefit from case management service."

Program Needs of Case Managers

Alternatives in a Rural Setting

In rural settings, agencies and professionals may simply lack the necessary prerequisites of a case management system. The agency may not have the funding or authority to purchase or authorize community care services, because local providers are funded with grants that do not give priority to the target population of the case management system. In such situations, there is less value to case management because the case management agency (and the consumers) is limited to the providers that are already funded to provide whatever services they chose, in whatever manner and at whatever cost they have negotiated with the funding source. At best, the case management agency may have a small amount of discretionary funding for gap-filling services. Lacking sufficient authority or resources, the agency cannot develop the highly individualized service plans necessary for high-risk clients. In other words, they can do assessments and offer good advice, but they cannot deliver a care plan.

In this situation, the best option may be to emphasize the advice-giving and problem-solving aspects of the service agency by focusing on a very effective information and assistance system with a strong outreach component. A good information and assistance service can assist consumers in locating the best available help for which they qualify or that they can afford. Once a referral to a provider is accomplished, however, ongoing monitoring becomes the responsibility of the service provider. Although invaluable, such programs lack systems of checks and balances; they are also not case management.

In addition, rural agencies that are well rooted in their communities can locate sources of informal support as well as formal providers, and may be able to stimulate the development of new resources through leadership in community planning and through informal contacts and networking. This approach is central to the national Eldercare Campaign initiated in 1991 by the federal Administration on Aging, which focuses on building community coalitions to expand resources to vulnerable elderly.

Ideally, the rural case manager should have the resources and authority to organize and purchase individualized services. For example, the most frequently used service in many rural areas is the individually employed generic home care worker (e.g., personal care attendant, chore worker, home care assistant). The case manager can arrange for the employment of neighbors and other local people to fill in the gaps where the certified Medicaid home health agency is unable to supply service.

Standards, Rules, Rights, and Restrictions

Inevitably, as states spend millions of dollars on case management in community care settings, standards are developed to assure quality and control costs. At the same time, professional organizations are developing their own standards for professional development of case managers. These general standards are written without regard to setting (rural or urban), yet are responsive to the unique circumstances of each.

The National Council on Aging

The National Council on Aging (NCOA) has developed generic standards for case management programs that apply to many models of case management. NCOA defines case management as a process to make the community care system work more effectively for individuals. The NCOA standards detail a philosophy of individual autonomy, recognizing the unique needs and preferences of individuals. Furthermore, the standards outline a defined target population, clients' rights, program goals, care managers roles, and program support functions such as training and evaluation. At the heart of the standards is a description of the elements of case management with some general qualitative statements about intake, assessment, care planning, service delivery, monitoring and reassessment, and discharge.

The NCOA standards call for uniform tools and adequate record keeping. They recommend that caseload size limitations be imposed by each program based on characteristics of the clients and the service system.

The National Association of Social Workers

The National Association of Social Workers (NASW) has standards and guidelines for social workers who do case management. Viewed less as program standards and more as a code of professional conduct, the NASW standards speak to issues of client self-determination, primacy of clients' interests versus agency interests, confidentiality, and interdisciplinary relationships. They call for advocacy on the part of the case manager, and they recognize the role of the family.

Development at the State Level

Washington, Oregon, and Pennsylvania are among the states that have well-developed standards for case management. These standards include guidance about how quickly consumers must be able to get into the service delivery system, how many clients can be managed by one case manager, and the required training and qualifications of case managers. Increasingly, states are developing standards that comply with requirements of the Title XIX (Medicaid) Home and Community Care Waiver programs. Some states, such as Wisconsin, are moving from program guidelines (which apply to the process of case management) toward standards for the tasks performed by each case manager.

In general, these standards address the activities of a single case manager (usually a social worker or nurse) who performs all the core tasks of case management. The assumption is that a multidisciplinary assessment process will occur, but the case manager is one individual with a relationship with the client that extends, as much as possible, through the processes of case management. The commonly accepted standards do conflict with the newly emerging industrial model of human service management, in which all clients pass through various units of a department that services many populations, with different units responsible for intake, eligibility screening, assessment, contracting for service, monitoring, and follow-along. Although many agencies call this series of administrative processes case management, the use of the term may be misleading, because it lacks the individual, client-centered approach that gives value to case management. Neither should this assembly-line approach be confused with multidisciplinary team approaches to case management, in which one key worker is the lead person on a team of professionals who all have roles in assisting a client—a complex version of case management that is unlikely to exist in rural areas outside of hospital or institutional settings.

Resource Management

The purpose of case management in any setting is to use resources more effectively to meet the needs of clients in a manner and setting that they prefer. Case managers are not direct service providers, although in many rural areas case managers do provide hands-on services because no one else is available. There are strong reasons, foremost of which is conflict of interest, they should not be employed by direct service providers.

The case manager requires a thorough knowledge of the formal services available in the community as well as the voluntary resources. This means knowledge of the hours of service, the competence of the providers, the geographic areas served, and their responsiveness to unique requests. Based on the knowledge of the client that develops through the assessment and care planning process, the case manager should be able to make very specific requests for service. Because many clients prefer home care services to be rendered in the morning, scheduling to meet these preferences may conflict with staffing patterns of agencies. If the case manager can develop a cooperative relationship with the agencies, it may be possible to convey some of the specific service issues and work out compatible solutions. For example, the agency may be able to schedule its workers for earlier morning hours (ending the workday earlier) and schedule all staff meetings and administrative tasks for the afternoons. A service provider might be able to recruit workers from a particular geographic area to reduce travel time. Availability of a desktop computer and modem may allow a worker to do some work at home rather than travel to an office each day.

The case manager has a unique overview of the client's needs and the services required. Coordination of the services of various providers can avoid duplication of, as well as gaps in, coverage. For example, if a client simply needs someone to check on him or her in person each day for security reasons (as in the case of someone with a high risk of falling), arrangements to schedule at least one provider visit each day, including volunteers and mobile meals, can be made. The role of each provider will include checking on the person's well-being and communicating that information to either the case manager or a lead provider agency designated by the case manager.

It is more often necessary to make service arrangements with the overall cost of the care plan in mind. For example, an assessment might suggest that an individual needs personal care and nutritional services several days each week, as well as a home-delivered meal on other days. If the costs of transporting that person to day care are excessive because of its location, and meal delivery also has high transport costs, it may be preferable to substitute a locally recruited home care worker who will prepare a meal, help with personal care, and assist the client with routine therapy (after receiving adequate training). The worker may actually be paid to play a game of cards or just visit for half an hour if the purpose of the day care included socialization.

Case management, especially in rural areas, requires that the case manager have the flexibility to use funding in the most cost-effective ways. That may include combining several program needs into a creative service option. In all cases, it is important that the case manager inform all service providers about what other service providers are doing with a given client, to avoid unnecessary duplication.

Many states currently have case management programs in various stages of development. An excellent resource regarding the state of the art in case management is the Center for the Advancement of State Community Care Programs, housed with the National Association of State Units on Aging (NASUA) in Washington, D.C. Information about how to contact NASUA can be obtained through any state unit on aging.

Among the states with highly developed programs are Washington and Oregon. After 10 years of managing targeted case management programs, both states have achieved a remarkable balance between the resources available for community care and for nursing home care. Washington's program is a real continuum, with access through an information and assistance (I&A) program. I&A workers screen clients at intake and make referrals either directly to providers or to case managers for assessment. The Oregon program is focused more directly on preadmission screening for persons seeking admission to nursing homes. Many clients who are assessed as needing nursing home care are successfully referred to an extensive network of assisted living arrangements, where case plans are implemented by residential providers.

Pennsylvania has been a pioneer in the development of "service management" through Area Agencies on Aging (AAAs). This original service has been expanded to provide a more intensive level of case management for clients identified in the preadmission screening program.

Although Wisconsin does not operate a preadmission screening program, it does restrict its Community Options Program to persons of any age who qualify for nursing home admission. The Community Options Program operates from a very flexible funding source that permits case managers to allow payment for anything identified in the assessment/care planning process, including home modifications and payments to relatives. As a primarily rural state, Wisconsin has made extensive use of locally recruited home care attendants, who may be employed by the client (who receives a cash payment for the purchase of care) or by an agency that places workers.

All of these states have been successful in serving a very disabled population for much less than the average cost of nursing home care for similar populations. Case managers are able to arrange higher-cost care packages provided that the average cost of care remains within the target. Earlier research, especially the National Channelling Demonstrations, failed to document the same cost savings (Haskins, Capitman, et al., 1985). States have learned from the failures of the early demonstrations, and have improved targeting and budget caps to ensure that costs are controlled.

While states have been developing policy and budget approaches to case management, Area Agencies on Aging have been carving out a role for AAAs as case management agencies in many places (including Oregon, Washington, Pennsylvania, Maine, and many other exemplary states). The National Association of Area Agencies on Aging has promoted standards, training, and legislation to advance the role of AAAs in this field.

Policy and Applied Research of Case Management

Policy

Politics and direct service delivery have always been at odds, especially because of the private agendas and opposing goals of individuals and agencies. Too often those responsible for the final program have only a cursory understanding of the realities and the needs of supervisors and case managers who are responsible for service delivery.

A Central Issue

A fundamental community-based long-term care policy debate central to case management, and one made critical for rural case management, is this: Given the often service poor environment, would the money spent in developing, implementing, and administering case management programs be better spent in developing comprehensive rural services? Analogous to the chicken and the egg debate, which should be developed first? Granted, services are essential, but without any coordinating element, such as case management, their effectiveness can often be seriously diminished. Services by themselves are insubstantial; it is only when they are accessible and appropriately allocated to those in need that they become meaningful.

Policy in Practice

At the policy level a state agency (or legislative body) awards the funds and therefore determines individual eligibility. In order to accomplish a stated public policy goal, state-funded home care or Medicaid home and community care waiver programs that offer case management services may define the client. Occasionally, the local AAA or a county social services department has the authority to plan for Older Americans Act or Social Services Block Grant home care programs within a service area, in which case target client populations are then determined locally. Target populations may be defined in terms of income and/or disability.

If the main goal of case management is the coordination of services in order to deliver assistance efficiently to keep someone at home, case management will benefit certain types of clients, specifically, persons with complex needs requiring multiple services/agencies/funding sources and persons lacking informal supports who cannot understand or negotiate the application for assistance in a complex system.

The service coordination model of case management can reduce duplication of services and provide access to help. It has not, however, proven generally cost-effective in controlled studies. That is, it does not necessarily save money, although it is generally accepted that the service coordination/case management approach improves the effectiveness of services through monitoring and personal contacts.

In rural areas, service agencies are scarce, therefore case managers may actually coordinate very few services. Furthermore, it is possible that some effective results may be achieved by employing a simpler system of outreach, information, and assistance. Intensive case management efforts are not necessary in cases where the main issues are helping people to find out what is available and helping them make application for assistance.

Community

Case management, as defined here, is not simple service coordination, but a process that operates in a community care system organized to achieve personal goals for the client and policy goals for the payer. For the client, the goals may include individually packaged services to meet personal needs and preferences, perhaps even tailoring existing services to "fit" unique circumstances. For the payer, whether the individual or the government, the goal may be limiting cost. To limit costs, it is necessary (a) to provide no more care than is necessary, (b) to limit the costs of providers, and (c) to make the best use of paraprofessional and voluntary support.

Why Case Management?

Case managers are important to older persons who want care at home or in the community because they can offer good advice. They can produce packages of services that respond to individuals' needs and preferences.

Despite the assertive word *manager,* the professional is really an adviser, and ultimately the older person is the one who should choose whether to accept the advice. The advice provided by a case manager is based on professional judgment as well as a thorough knowledge of the client's strengths and resources, as well as the deficiencies in the client's abilities and environment. Client information is collected through a process of assessment based on observation and interviewing. Once the case manager and the client have identified and agreed upon the services required, the critical challenge is to determine how to meet those needs within the limits of the community where the client resides. That means arranging for service providers and home modifications, and determining the cost of a package of care.

Authority

Case managers are most likely to be effective at meeting client needs for appropriate services, and the policy goals of containing cost, if they have the authority to arrange payment for services and to influence the cost of service. Service providers may be more flexible in adjusting schedules or in agreeing to perform specialized tasks for an agency that controls at least part of their payment. If the case manager is only a coordinator of services, or broker, he or she is forced to rely solely on persuasion to obtain appropriate services. Furthermore, when a case manager controls at least part of the funding source, he or she may be able to purchase "gap-filling" services to plug the holes in the existing array of services. With at least some resources at his or her disposal, the case manager may be able to leverage provision of a service that does not currently exist, such as off-hours or weekend help.

In a well-developed system, the case manager can provide a range of options in care planning to enable the consumer to choose the most acceptable manner of receiving help. For example, the consumer can choose between a daytime companion or transport to day care certain days of the week. The case manager will also cost out the approximate price of the care plan, to determine the most cost-effective arrangement. Whether the individual or the government is paying (or funding is coming from a combination of sources), all payers will be more supportive of the case manager's role if it includes cost-conscious management of resources.

Another role of the case manager in a system of community care is that of a gatekeeper. Because resources are limited, services cannot be provided on demand. The case manager is responsible for determining who has first claim on the resources. Policies of the agency or funding source should lay out the criteria or priorities for admitting a client to the system; the case manager then uses his or her judgment in deciding whether a client fits the criteria. Because case managers are such key players in the system, their informed opinions should be considered in making such policies. In many instances, case managers become advocates for clients, working to bring about changes in policies that are unnecessarily exclusionary or unfairly vague or arbitrary.

Finally, the case manager has a quality improvement role. By regular monitoring on the phone and in person, the case manager can determine whether the needs and preferences of the consumer are being met, and can initiate changes in the care arrangements or daily routine to increase satisfaction.

Research Issues

To date, much of the body of work on case management has been theoretical or has concentrated on specific programs, such as the Robert Woods Johnson Foundation Program for Hospital Initiatives in Long-Term Care. Larger-scale investigations such as that conducted by Krout (1991a) have been limited to obtaining cursory descriptive data. Although these efforts are laudable, more are needed. Future studies should focus on adding to the qualitative body of knowledge regarding case management, with an emphasis on understanding case management as it is practiced on a wide scale and answering the following questions: What is interpreted as case management? What does it actually do and for whom? How is it perceived by case managers, supervisors, and policy makers? Most important, how can we provide what in theory works so well, but falls short of its potential in practice?

Many additional research questions concern program execution and policy, such as the following: Exactly how much latitude in purchasing services can administrators and supervisors allow? How can case management programs foster innovation and creativity in care planning? How can case managers merge cost consciousness with effective care plans? How do programmers evaluate the working environment to develop a "best fit" case management service?

Many of these issues are directly related to training. It may be that training in creative management techniques, fostering empowerment, and utilizing basic budgeting skills, by providing cost information at the primary level of the case manager, could help develop the potential of case management. The guidelines and standards exists—it is the level of execution that is lacking. We need to begin treating the existing standards as minimums that must be attained instead of viewing them as maximums. Guidelines and standards are necessary to establish community expectations as to what constitutes case management—what should be paid for, and what should not. The establishment of some community expectations will help to protect vulnerable individuals (such as the elderly and their families) from private, unscrupulous exploiters.

In addition, we need to conduct research into the direct outcomes of case management intervention, both the tangibles and the intangibles. Some early work has been completed (Capitman, Haskins, & Bernstein, 1986; Eggert, 1986; Secord, 1987), but, given the recent strides in and evolution of case management, this area needs review and evaluation. Research is needed on a national scale, with a variety of programs participating. It may be that the real value of such studies would be in enabling us to define the intangible benefits of case management. Finally, the key research issue is how to assure that those individuals most in need of case management receive services.

Summary

Case management is a tool used by policy makers, strategic planners, and fieldworkers. Its elemental contribution to strategic planning is the crucial investment of time and energy that every program needs in order to conduct "fire prevention." It counters the argument, often heard in rural areas, that an agency does not have the luxury of time for planning by saying, in effect, neither do you have the time to fail.

In both rural and urban areas the case management process has the capacity to cross lines and to coordinate both clinical care and administrative procedures, working as both a cost management mechanism and a coordinating tool for local community and state programs, as well as for federally subsidized programs.

When utilized to its fullest capacity, case management can effectively address issues of community cooperation, staffing, and the flexibility of funding streams (putting the money where it will do the most good). If the process confines creativity or blocks open communication between any of the agencies or individuals involved, then some crucial element is missing, or the philosophical intent behind its mission has been overlooked or forgotten.

Overall, but most important in rural areas, there is a need for basic consistency and uniformity in the understanding of the potential of case management. Those who pay the bills, those who provide care, and those who receive care can only benefit through achieving consensus on the responsibilities and expectations of a program. Agencies and state and area planners must define the expected role and expected outcomes of case management in the long-term care continuum.

In addition, consensus among community organizations is needed in each program to identify target populations. The responsibility of deciding who will or will not gain access to services is a policy question. Rural agencies offering case management services need to foster both formal and informal interagency communications to facilitate client access to services and to minimize red tape. Additionally, agencies need to institute some form of consistent and uniform training for all case managers. Case managers are individuals who can think, create, and care. They understand the big picture—that is, they understand the ramifications and consequences of their actions on both clinical and administrative levels. Given the demographics of rural areas, area planners and agencies have a unique opportunity to create integrated systems of service delivery. The strengths of rural agencies coupled with well-communicated case management guidelines for expected outcomes can only work toward better fulfilling the needs of the rural elderly.

5

Senior Centers
in Rural Communities

JOHN A. KROUT
MARGARET M. WILLIAMS
OLLIE OWEN

One of the biggest gaps in the gerontological and senior center literature is the paucity of information on the nature, roles, and activities of senior centers in *rural* communities. This lack of research persists despite the recognition of the important roles played by senior centers and constitutes a significant gap in our understanding of both senior centers and rural environments (for a complete review of the senior center literature, see Krout, 1989c). Indeed, the need for a clear understanding of successful rural senior centers is manifest, as gerontological research has consistently shown rural areas to have fewer services for the elderly than do nonrural areas (Coward & Lee, 1985a; Krout, 1986, 1989a). Because service providers and sites are generally lacking in rural areas, senior centers are often the *only* service/information and referral points for elders in those areas and also serve as a key link to the larger health and human services network (Krout, 1989c, 1992). Senior centers can take on particular importance as a focal point for providing supportive services to older persons living in isolated rural areas.

Thus there is a critical need for more information on how rural senior centers successfully support programming and provide services, and how the problems faced by rural senior center staff can be overcome. Further, as noted in Chapter 1 of this volume, rural elders are generally found to have higher levels of need in areas such as income, housing, health, and transportation. Rural senior centers can serve as resources for the entire community as well as the elderly, and can provide opportunities for community members to empower themselves and their communities. Rural centers provide opportunities for rural elders not only to receive services and social support, but also to contribute their knowledge and leadership skills.

In this chapter we provide an overview of rural senior center organizational, programming, and participant characteristics. We then identify key considerations that rural center practitioners, advocates, planners, and volunteers need to keep in mind when assessing center activities, as well as fundamental elements of senior center success. We also provide specific examples of how rural senior centers have thrived in the face of various difficulties, and offer a discussion of central research and policy issues affecting rural senior centers.

Senior Center Overview

Recent estimates place the number of senior centers in this country at about 10,000 (Krout, 1989c; Schulder, 1985). Many senior centers provide a wide range of health, social, recreational, and educational services (Krout, 1985) and are the most frequently used service delivery sites and designated focal points established by Area Agencies on Aging (AAAs) (Krout, 1989a). Senior centers are well known to older persons (Krout, 1984a; Leanse & Wagner, 1975) and research has shown that between 15% and 20% of the elderly in this country participate in senior center activities (Louis Harris and Associates, 1975; Krout, 1989c). Research on who among the elderly participate in senior centers is equivocal, with findings often related to the nature of the particular center studied (Krout, 1989c). Krout, Cutler, and Coward (1990) analyzed data from a large national sample of almost 14,000 elderly, and found that senior center users, compared with nonusers, in general, were more likely to be female, to live alone, and to reside in suburban and rural nonfarm areas. They also had lower incomes and fewer problems with activities of daily living, but higher levels of social interaction than seniors who do not use centers. Age and education were related to center participation in a curvilinear fashion; race and self-reported health status were unrelated to center use.

The general lack of availability and accessibility of rural services would suggest lower utilization rates for rural centers. However, research findings on this issue have been equivocal. May, Herrman, and Fitzgerald (1976) found no rural/urban differences for participation in a congregate meal program, and Taietz (1970) found considerably higher senior center attendance rates in a New York State study for a sample of rural versus urban older persons. Recent analysis of a large national data set by Krout et al. (1990) reveals an interesting pattern for community size differences in senior center utilization. These researchers found similar overall utilization rates for nonmetropolitan nonfarm residents (15%) and suburban elderly (14%), and a slightly lower rate for central-city elders (12%). Only 8% of elderly farm dwellers, on the other hand, reported using senior centers. The relatively high rates for nonmetropolitan nonfarm elders may reflect a higher level of need for services and a greater availability of senior centers, whereas the lower rates for farm dwellers may reflect availability and accessibility problems and the greater availability of spousal support, because older farm residents are more likely than nonfarm dwellers to be married (Krout, 1986).

Previous research suggests that a sizable number of senior centers can be found in rural areas across the United States. Perhaps the first comprehensive, national study of senior centers that provided some attention to the rural scene was conducted in the early 1970s by the National Council on the Aging (Leanse & Wagner, 1975). This study collected survey data from nearly 5,000 senior centers and clubs. Of the senior centers, only 23% indicated that they were located in "rural" places (59% said urban, 16% said suburban, and 2% were not classified). It is very likely that response rate differences by location and bias in the master listing used in the study contributed to this low rural presence. It is also quite possible that relatively few rural communities had senior centers in place two decades ago. Indeed, Krout (1983), in a study using a 1982 National Council on the Aging senior center list, found that one-half of the 4,000 centers from the 33 state listings were located in nonmetropolitan counties. Sela (1986), on the other hand, reports that 32% of some 6,000 senior centers responding to a nationwide survey focusing on center participation of the hearing impaired were rural.

National surveys conducted in the 1970s and 1980s found that rural senior centers, compared with urban centers, have lower budgets, smaller numbers of volunteer and paid staff, and smaller numbers of activities and services. Their facilities are smaller and more likely to be in one-story buildings (Krout, 1983; Leanse & Wagner, 1975), and they are more likely to be part of Area Agencies on Aging (Krout, 1983). Some of the rural/urban differences are considerable. For example, Krout's 1982 study of more than 600 senior centers in 33 states found that 42% of the most rural centers reported annual budgets of less than $10,000, whereas a similar percentage of the most urban centers reported budgets of $75,000 and above (Krout, 1984b, 1987). Krout (1990b) resurveyed this sample in 1989 to uncover changes it had experienced during the 1980s. Compared with the urban centers, the rural centers were less likely to report increases in programming, budgets, and participation. More variation was found for the rural than the urban centers, and whereas most urban centers expanded in these areas, the rural centers could be about evenly classified into three groups; decliners, maintainers, and expanders.

However, it is important to note that even though rural senior centers support a smaller number of activities and services than urban centers, they still offer a wide range of programming. Krout's longitudinal study of senior centers found that even centers in communities of fewer than 2,500 persons reported offering, on average, 15 services and activities in 1989. Senior centers located in places of population 50,000 or more reported an average of 22 services and activities (Krout, 1990b). A majority of rural senior centers reportedly offer information and referral, health screening and education, recreation, socialization, congregate and in-home meals, and nutrition education (Krout, 1990b). Centers in smaller communities offer these programs less frequently, however, and the depth and breadth of programming offered under each activity and service heading may be less than is found in more urban centers.

The participants of the rural centers in 1989 were somewhat older and poorer and more likely to be white than for urban centers. In addition, it would appear that rural centers were more likely to have experienced an "aging in place" of participants during the 1980s, as rural directors were more likely to report that their user populations had gotten older. Rural respondents were also less likely to report increases in the income and health status of center participants (Krout, 1990b). These data suggest that rural center users are in greater need of a large array of income support programs (e.g., SSI, food stamps, home heating assistance, tax reductions, and income supplement opportunities) that senior centers could provide or assist participants to identify and become involved with through education and referral activities. Health and wellness education and promotion (e.g., nutrition, exercise, stress reduction, drugs) as well as a wide variety of regularly scheduled health screening activities (dental, blood pressure, vision, diet, diabetes) also appear to be particularly salient for rural center populations.

Unfortunately, many of the program needs noted above are generally less likely to be adequately met in rural areas, because senior centers and the aging services network in general lack the dollars and health service professionals to provide them. However, this does not mean that those program needs are impossible to fill, only that filling them is more challenging. Training and resource materials can and should be developed to fit the needs of rural center participants and build the capacity of rural centers to meet them. Finally, traditional linkages with other agencies and the adoption of communication technology (e.g., remote broadcast and videos) can also serve to overcome resource gaps and accessibility problems.

To summarize, the data indicate considerable variation among rural centers and suggest that the stereotype of the dying rural senior center is indeed overdrawn. Given the overall lack of services in rural areas, senior centers would appear to be a crucial link in providing social, recreational, educational, and health services to rural elders. We now turn to an examination of the fundamental dimensions by which rural senior centers can be measured.

Basic Dimensions of Rural Senior Centers

It is difficult and even inappropriate to generalize about rural centers, because variety seems to be their defining characteristic. Nonetheless, generalizations are required to develop an overall understanding of the different ways in which they perform basic senior center functions. Traditionally, senior centers in rural areas are located in separate *facilities* (often one or two main rooms and bathroom facilities). Sometimes they utilize space in community centers, churches, or even fire halls, but centers without their own facilities often serve largely as nutrition sites. Facilities can be categorized in two ways: those adapted for the use of the program but whose primary purpose is other than use as a senior center (i.e., churches, American Legion halls, Grange halls) and those that have been built or remodeled for the purpose of housing a senior center. Generally speaking, the former type of facility is less adequate for programming purposes (see Krout, 1988a).

The *nutrition* (or congregate/in-home meal) function is very important for all rural senior centers and often serves as an anchor for other programming. Many times this other programming consists of socialization, recreation (card playing, bingo, trips), and education on a range of health, legal, and self-improvement issues. It is important to recognize that many rural elders attend centers mainly for the social and recreational (and volunteering) opportunities and because the centers serve as "communities" that provide them with a sense of integration with others (Krout, 1988b). Some rural centers have much wider and more sophisticated ranges of programming that require more professional staff skills and linkages with other agency personnel. Programming can be categorized as ranging from largely *single purpose,* such as nutrition and/or recreation, to *multipurpose,* intended to meet a larger diversity of needs and participants, including seniors with physical, cognitive, or economic loses. The nature of facilities and the array of programming make up two dimensions by which rural senior centers can be characterized.

Both of these dimensions are closely related to the availability of financial resources and professional staff, two other important dimensions. Rural center budgets range from almost nothing to hundreds of thousands of dollars, and staff can vary from all volunteer or half full-time equivalent to full-time college-educated directors accompanied by staff devoted to social activities, outreach, transportation, nutrition, volunteers, and so on (Krout, 1987, 1992). Thus budgets range from *bare bones* to *resource rich,* and staffing patterns from *all volunteer* to *multiprofessional.* In addition to staffing patterns, the roles played by participants in planning, implementing, and revising center programming are also an important element in determining participation patterns. Participant involvement in center operation can range from virtually nonexistent, suggesting a *nonparticipatory* form of authority structure, where decisions are made by staff alone or by a very small clique of participants, to a *pluralistic democratic* authority structure, where decision making is shared by staff and participants.

Another dimension has to do with where the senior center fits within the larger aging network. Some rural centers are closely connected administratively and through planning and funding to AAAs; others function with minimal contact with these organizations (Krout, 1989a). The *focal-point* function is an important aspect of this dimension. Some rural senior centers have a fairly high degree of interaction, through referral and other activities, with AAAs, hospitals, home health agencies, legal services, and other components of the community-based care system. These centers are often designated as official focal points by local Area Agencies on Aging. They can benefit from mutual marketing, referral of potential participants, and funding for services. These factors enhance the center's ability to attract a wider variety of seniors and to provide a wider variety of programming. Other rural centers are fairly self-contained and have limited contact with such organizations. For example, senior centers in Wyoming (by many standards the most rural state in the country) serve as the home base for the state's case management system and thus act as a funnel through which seniors are directed to services allocated under that program. The Nebraska Department on Aging has developed a process by which rural senior centers work with an array of community interest groups to serve as focal points for community service development, not just for the elderly.

Although the degree of interaction with other agencies can be heavily influenced by factors such as financial and staff resources, terrain, population density, and availability of and distance to service providers, it also reflects the orientation of center staff and participants. A rural center that is fairly isolated in terms of distance and terrain need not be isolated from other community-based services. Thus rural senior centers can range from playing almost no focal-point roles and being *atomistic* or uninvolved with other organizations to serving as central service and information/referral *focal points*.

The importance of adequate and affordable transportation for seniors to centers in rural areas cannot be stressed enough. Whether this transportation is provided by seniors themselves, relatives, friends, or neighbors or by transportation programs funded by federal, state, and/or local dollars, it is essential for the survival of a congregate program such as a senior center. Generally, successful senior centers are integrated with or even directly provide transportation systems of one kind or another. Affordable and convenient *access* to rural senior centers is a necessity for success. Centers unable to provide transportation in one form or another to rural seniors are unlikely to prosper.

Finally, some rural centers serve as hubs for networks of satellite centers or nutrition sites and play significant resource and coordinating functions for those networks. In other areas, each rural community has a senior center that functions independently in terms of funding and administration and pretty much replicates the programming of centers found in other communities. Thus this dimension ranges from the *hub-and-spoke* to the *single- or multiple-hub* arrangement.

To sum up, rural senior center approaches can be distinguished on the basis of a number of dimensions, several of which have been identified here: facilities, programming, budget, staffing, participant involvement, access, focal-point status, and hub status. Many other dimensions could be identified, but these eight are seen as basic to other rural senior center issues. Rural senior centers that fall on different points of each dimension, singularly and in combination, can all be effective and provide appropriate responses to the needs of rural elders. No one combination is necessarily best. Clearly, rural centers with larger facilities that are resource rich, that have professional staff and serve as focal points within a hub-and-spoke arrangement, are likely in a position to serve a larger number of rural elders with an array of service needs ranging from recreation to adult day services. Generally speaking, however, the research reviewed in the first section of this chapter suggests that most rural senior centers do not have all of these characteristics. We now turn to a discussion of the fundamental issues and questions that must be addressed in order for rural senior centers to be successful.

Fundamentals for
Successful Rural Center Programming

In general, rural senior centers, like senior centers in other community settings, must address a number of issues and barriers to develop and maintain effective programming for elders. One way to identify and organize these issues is the use of the "five A's" formula discussed by Krout (1986) and Williams, Ebrite, and Redford (1991). The A's are as follows:

- *accessibility*
  Is the program or service accessible to rural elders?
  Do the elderly feel comfortable entering the program?
  Are service agencies aware of the program and do they refer clients to it?
  Are staff knowledgeable, trained, and caring? Are they prepared to assist rural elders?

- *affordability*

  Are the programs affordable given the level of financial resources of the rural elders in the area?

  Are mechanisms in place to secure payment for the program, such as voluntary contributions or fees?

- *appropriateness*

  Will the service provide programs that are needed and wanted by older persons in the area?

  Do programs take into account the rural elderly's personal preferences?

- *adequacy*

  Is the program designed to allow persons to enter at the levels they need, not offering too little or too much?

  Does the program enable individuals to remain independent for as long as possible?

  Does the program meet persons' minimal needs?

- *acceptability*

  Is the program in sync with the attitudes, values, and beliefs of the rural elderly to be served?

  Will the personnel providing the programs be acceptable to the rural elderly?

  Will the services meet older persons' needs as those persons define them?

Successful rural senior centers do not just happen, nor can all rural centers necessarily be considered successful simply because they are in operation. Careful attention must be paid to the five A's (they must be addressed and readdressed) and to developing a plan that will guide the expenditure of resources in the short and long term. The most important of the five A's for the senior center is *acceptability.* If center programming is not acceptable to the target population, the programs will not succeed. Senior center staff and "consumers" must identify goals for the center and develop a plan to accomplish those goals. At the most basic level, such a plan should address the areas of *what, how, who, where, when,* and *why* in regard to center activities.

- *What* is it that you want to accomplish (goals)?

  Services or a one-stop referral/focal point?

  Meals? Education? Raise income?

Opportunities to volunteer?

Opportunities to return something to the community?

- *How* will this be done?

How and where will the funding be found?

How will the staff be found and trained?

How will the programs be marketed?

How will the services be provided?

- *Who* will be involved?

Who is it that the senior center wants to serve? That is, who are the targeted elderly?

Who will raise the funds needed?

Who will conduct the programs?

Who should be on the boards?

Who should be on the planning committees?

Who will staff the senior center?

- *Where* will the services be provided?

What town and site?

Can people get to the site?

Are there facilities available or will they have to be built?

Are the facilities accessible to physically challenged elders?

- *When* will the senior center be open?

What days and hours will it be open?

- *Why* are particular programs being provided?

Do the programs meet the needs of a variety of people?

Can the programs be done well?

Is there involvement in and ownership of the programs by the participants?

Are the staff interacting with the participants in a productive way?

These basic questions are too often ignored or addressed informally, without adequate time or energy from staff or input from center users and other community constituencies, especially older persons who do not utilize senior centers. To be fair, many center staff and volunteers in rural areas simply lack the time and resources to conduct systematic evaluations of center goals and activities. We would suggest, however, that despite limitations in these and other areas, those involved in operating rural senior centers *must* address these questions.

Guidelines for
Successful Rural Senior Center Operation

The senior author of this chapter recently completed an examination of activities that are fundamental to the operation of successful congregate programs (Krout, 1991c). This examination did not focus on rural senior centers per se, but it seems to have considerable applicability to this topic. These fundamentals do not necessarily require a lot of money, but they do require a considerable investment of time and a commitment to examining every facet of a senior center's operation. Nothing can be held sacred. The areas covered include goals and identity, image and marketing, community roles, programming, access and facilities, planning and evaluation, and running a center. The recommendations for each of these areas are presented below.

Goals and Identity

- Clear goals help form a program identity.
- Goals should have specific objectives attached to them, so success can be defined and measured.
- Goal statements should be drawn up by advisory boards and informed by participants.
- Goal statements are helpful in attracting community support as well as new participants.
- The goal development process can help to identify differences in opinions held by board members and/or participants.

Image and Marketing

- Senior center staff should have a good idea of the program's image in the community.
- Staff should have a plan in place to create a specific image through use of mass media, fund-raising, programming, and so on.
- The name of a senior center can play a big part in its image.
- Staff should consciously work on "selling" programs and should understand the "costs" to participants and trade-offs they make when they choose to participate.
- Special attention should be given to "first contact" personnel, but even custodial staff affect the tone of the program.

Community Roles, Linkages, and Focal Points

- The roles played by a senior center should be recognized and understood by program staff.
- Community roles should be established and visible.
- Linkages with a wide range of organizations and groups in the community should be planned, instituted, and assessed.
- A process designed to build linkages with a broad-based coalition of community interest groups is important and beneficial.
- Senior centers should strive to act as community focal points for elderly services.

Running a Congregate Program

Senior center staff should take on the following responsibilities:

- Foster and encourage participant involvement in program planning and operation.
- Establish a climate as well as mechanisms and structures for such involvement (e.g., advisory board committee membership).
- Allow for broad-based participant involvement.
- Provide information on participant responsibilities and rights.
- Foster a sense of program ownership among participants.
- Relate to the needs and concerns of participants.
- Demonstrate good interpersonal and leadership skills.
- Be flexible and creative in working with participants and developing programs.

In addition, senior staff should be afforded opportunities for training, self-improvement, and professional advancement.

Senior center directors should do the following:

- Show respect for participants and staff and a sincere enjoyment of their position.
- Avoid becoming or appearing too close to some participants (or staff) as opposed to others.
- Show leadership in all areas while delegating tasks to others where appropriate.
- Be in control while providing for input from participants and staff.

Also, as for senior staff, directors should be treated as professionals, and should be afforded opportunities for training and self-improvement.

Advisory boards serve multiple functions in support of congregate programs and directors. Board members should reflect the demographic makeup of the community and program participants, and should include representatives from various institutions in the community. Effective advisory boards will do the following:

- Meet regularly and follow a written agenda.
- Have a number of committees that report regularly.
- Have a chair who keeps in close communication with congregate directors.

Those responsible for coordinating volunteers should be aware of several things:

- Volunteering provides program participants with opportunities for involvement and ownership.
- Volunteers can serve as very effective "public relations" personnel.
- Volunteer workers are not "free"; their involvement requires a lot of time and resources.
- Volunteers require specific guidelines and expectations about job performance, as well as evaluation and training.
- Successful retention of volunteers is dependent not only on recognition, but also on a careful recruitment and supervision process.

Programming

Programming is a key to the continued survival and growth of any congregate program. In the case of senior centers, it must be carefully planned to respond to the interests of a diverse older population. Those involved in programming can use it to do the following:

- Create new volunteer opportunities.
- Build on and uncover the talents of existing program users.
- Serve important public relations and fund-raising functions.

Program designers can also work to attract nonusers, by taking the following steps:

- Identify program goals and objectives.
- Assess information on the community's older population and target groups.
- Develop a "program grid" to determine the program interests of different groups.
- Develop programs to meet those interests, remembering that good programs do not necessarily cost a lot of money.
- Develop and implement a program assessment plan.

Facilities

- Facilities should meet all regulations concerning accessibility for persons with disabilities.
- Facilities should incorporate design and physical features as much as possible to be practical for and attractive to elders with sensory impairments.
- Attractive and spacious facilities and adequate parking contribute to the success of congregate programs, but can be outweighed by an unfriendly atmosphere.
- A modern, new facility, however, is neither sufficient nor even necessary for a successful program.
- Congregate facilities are competing with many attractive alternatives.
- Many improvements in facilities do not require major investments or changes.
- Facility improvement provides opportunities for participant, volunteer, and community involvement.

Access

- Congregate sites should be located in areas that are accessible and inviting.
- Transportation and safe escort to congregate sites are key elements in program success.
- Ride sharing and volunteer programs as well as the use of other transportation resources should be utilized and supported.

Planning and Evaluation

- Congregate programs should be guided by a planning process that establishes short- and long-term goals.
- Advisory boards are often a good vehicle through which to develop the planning process.

- Input on the planning process should be sought from staff, participants, and community interests, but planning is ultimately the director's responsibility.
- A plan should include goals and objectives as well as specific action steps that will be taken to meet them.
- Objectives should be specific and measurable, with data that are available or relatively easy to obtain.
- The plan should include methods or procedures that allow a determination of the quantitative and qualitative outcomes of programs.
- Planning and evaluation should be ongoing.

Innovative Rural Senior Center Approaches

A dearth of information is available on rural senior center programming. Thus it is difficult to state with certainty "what works" or how successful rural senior centers become successful. Many of the reasons for success (or failure) depend on the particular center, staff, and rural community. The evidence does seem to suggest that the days of rural senior centers thriving simply by offering a noon meal, opportunities for socialization, and infrequent activities are going, if not already gone. Neither the young-old nor program funders are satisfied with such a traditional and often uninspired approach. The rural centers that do survive and thrive will be those that aggressively position themselves to meet the needs of an increasingly diverse rural older population.

We are aware of a number of rural senior centers that have done things "differently" and created important niches for themselves in their communities and in the lives of older persons. These examples have been gleaned from presentations delivered at the annual conference of the National Council on the Aging. They clearly are only a few examples of what creative and energetic practitioners have been able to achieve in rural areas. They demonstrate that solid community linkages, aggressive marketing, and creative management can overcome the resource deficits often found in rural areas and can lead to successful senior center focal-point activities.

Buffalo Senior Center, Wyoming. This center is located in a community of 3,300 (Buffalo) in a county of slightly more than 6,000 persons covering more than 4,000 square miles. One-third of Buffalo's population is aged 60 or older. To support a nutrition program in such a rural area, the senior center has joined forces with four local banks. The banks support the (homemade) meals program with both money and personnel. Open 364 days a year, the center has become a true focal point, not just for older persons but for the entire community. It provides the only public transportation in the county and rents the center facility to other groups for multiple uses. The center elicits input from other organizations and interests groups through an "eldercare" council. Center staff are also aggressively involved in community efforts to attract retirees and vacationers to the area. In short, the center staff and participants see themselves as running not a senior center, but a business that is integral to the well-being of the entire community and region.

DeKalb County Council on Aging, Alabama. Faced with the loss of local government funding for eight rural senior centers in northern Alabama, the DeKalb County Council's director decided to fight rather than cut services. Located in an area that produces more socks than anywhere else in the world, the director looked for ways to benefit from this local industry. A not-for-profit corporation was formed that employs seniors to "pair and package" socks for local sock mills—a real "cottage industry." The program not only generates monies that support the rural senior centers, but also provides employment for older persons in an area where such opportunities are limited. It also has helped fund the construction of a new focal-point center in the largest community in the area. Many programs, involving nutrition, transportation, health education, and employment, are based at the new center. By creatively utilizing the resources available in the local area, this aging services organization was able to build and expand in the face of funding cutbacks.

Senior Resource Center, Evergreen, Colorado. This center is located in the mountains west of Denver and serves parts of three rural "range" counties. Transportation is a real challenge because of poor roads and heavy winter snowfalls. Using $30,000 in county funds as seed money, local aging network practitioners went to work fund-raising and built a senior center to provide comprehensive services to both active and vulnerable (especially isolated) older persons. Trained volunteers are used to provide as many services as possible to isolated vulnerable seniors through a case management program based at the senior center. A professional case manager recruits the volunteers from throughout the area and provides training and supervision of services. Without this arrangement, the isolated seniors would not be receiving any services at all.

Central Missouri Office for the Aging, Columbia, Missouri. This Area Agency on Aging serves 19 mostly rural counties. Over the years, attendance at the 35 local senior centers, especially in the congregate meal program, had fallen off significantly. The AAA director realized that these declines were threatening the viability of the centers and their role in service provision and information and referral. To reverse this trend, the director embarked on a program to renew the center's nutrition programs through cost containment, customer satisfaction, and community involvement. Changing to one primary vendor for raw food that also provided a centralized delivery and inventory system and a standardized 25-day cycle menu resulted in considerable savings, including no change in raw food costs for six years. This has allowed the agency to put more money into other programs. Meals are prepared on-site and individual centers have some flexibility in food preparation methods and menu choices.

To enhance customer satisfaction, the "reservation" system was ended and meal serving times expanded, allowing more choice and flexibility for seniors. Low-fat, low-cholesterol meals as well as menu choices were also introduced. These seemingly small changes resulted in a doubling in average daily meal attendance, including an increase in attendance among newly retired older persons and a virtual elimination of nutrition program complaints. Food that is prepared but not served is quickly frozen and then delivered by volunteers to isolated or homebound seniors. Thus, with creative thinking and tough management, the future of the 35 rural senior centers seems much more secure as attendance figures, revenues, and client satisfaction have all increased.

Using technology. Modern communications technology does hold considerable promise for programming in rural senior centers, if they can garner the resources to buy computers, printers, modems, VCRs, and fax machines. These machines can serve as the basis for establishing rural networks and linking rural centers with information sources regardless of their physical location. VCRs can be used for staff training and to bring all kinds of information to center participants. Indeed, an electronic community for older adults has been in operation since 1986. The Seniornet network started as a research project at the University of San Francisco, and exists as a not-for-profit organization that strives to teach computer skills to older adults. It now consists of 34 local sites and 3,500 individual members, including senior centers, where classes are offered in computer applications such as word processing, database management, spreadsheets, and telecommunications. The sites and independent members with their own computers are linked nationally by an on-line network allowing communication via electronic mail. Such a network can help minimize isolation and loneliness for rural elders.

Research and Policy Issues

Obviously, it becomes important for research, practice, and policy to determine the conditions or factors under which different rural center experiences unfold. Many alternative (and empirically untested) explanations for the relative lack of growth among the majority of rural senior centers reported earlier exist: Rural centers and rural center programming are less attractive to the new cohort of young-old; rural center user populations are "aging in place" and literally dying off; macrodemographic changes in rural communities over the past several decades have severely reduced the number of potential center users; resources for rural centers have dried up as a result of the general rural economic malaise; federal and state policies favor urban and suburban areas; and increases in the number of and targeting to more frail elders have led to a redirection of aging dollars away from centers to in-home supportive care (Krout, 1992).

Determining the relative importance of these factors in any given community will require costly and time-consuming research that senior centers have neither the resources nor the capabilities to do. It is imperative that gerontological researchers and funders develop a research agenda to ensure that these questions are investigated in a timely and appropriate manner. The factors noted above also illustrate the complex web within which rural senior centers must operate to meet the needs of a diverse population of elders. Policy makers, planners, and gerontological educators need to recognize these complexities as they formulate programmatic and reimbursement requirements.

There is a need for research on virtually all aspects of rural senior center operation, programming, participation patterns, and participant characteristics. Who uses or does not use rural centers and why? What impact does center participation have on older persons? How are "at-risk" older persons best served by rural centers? What kinds of focal-point functions can and do rural senior centers play? What are the costs and benefits of rural senior centers for individuals, the aging services network, and communities? What resources are needed to provide a minimum of effective programming? What, if any, minimum level of programming should rural senior centers provide? What types of center programming are most effective? What kinds of training and technical assistance are most needed by rural center professional staff and volunteers? How is this assistance best provided? What roles can and do volunteers play in rural senior centers? How can rural centers serve nonelderly rural populations in need? Data on all these topics and more are needed. Little is known about the variability in rural center operation and successful or unsuccessful programming.

On a more practical level, it is important to note that rural senior centers need to be looked at carefully and objectively in regard to many questions if they are to be successful. A clear vision and statement of goals and objectives are fundamental to successful rural center operation. Basic questions must be asked and answered, but always with the recognition that resources, programming, and population characteristics and needs change continually and require flexible, creative, and quick responses. What needs and for whom among the elderly or the community do senior centers hope to address? What are the target populations? What do the elderly in the community want, and what services provided in what ways are they likely to find acceptable? What resources can reasonably be expected to be available for programming, staff, and facilities? What kind of programming has worked or failed in the past? What kind of education is required to change attitudes that resist needed and appropriate change?

Many of these questions presuppose consensus on basic policy issues for which such consensus either has not been reached or, more likely, has not even been attempted. Many rural service priorities and goals have gained their visibility through default, because other options have not been carefully explored. In some rural areas, the role of senior centers in serving older populations is well recognized and known; in other places it is not. Indeed, what should be the roles of rural senior centers in the aging social and health care network? To what degree should frail and other at-risk older persons be accommodated by general center programs and operations? What roles should rural senior centers play in intergenerational programming? What should be role of the centers in rural communities (economically and socially)? What do rural senior centers do better than others and could/should they be significantly changed? What portion of public dollars should they receive?

A careful consideration and resolution of these issues based on input from rural older persons and practitioners is needed if the quantity and quality of services for rural older persons are to improve significantly.

Finally, we must recognize that the challenges facing rural senior centers will only increase in the future. These challenges include funding, attracting the young-old, programming/integrating the frail, issues of center efficacy and creativity, volunteers and leadership, medicalization of services, and cost containment.

Summary and Conclusions

Senior centers in many rural communities play multifaceted and important roles in providing supportive activities and services to older persons. Their importance in this regard is multiplied by the general lack of availability of health and human services in rural areas and problems in accessing services. Rural senior centers can serve as local focal points for information and referral, providers of a wide range of services, and links to specialized services not provided locally. Despite this, the existing research on rural senior centers is minuscule; a critical need exists for more information on their operation and effectiveness, successful rural center program models, and strategies that can be employed to overcome the many problems and challenges they face.

This chapter has provided an overview of the basic elements of rural senior center operation and programming. We have argued that rural senior centers, like other components of the community-based long-term care system, must successfully address issues that can be categorized as relating to accessibility, affordability, appropriateness, adequacy, and acceptability. We have also provided a listing of basic activities and principles seen as fundamental to the success of senior center programs. They are meant to serve as guidelines for practitioners as they seek to improve existing or to develop new congregate programming and include goals and identity, image and marketing, community roles, programming, access and facilities, planning and evaluation, and running a center.

There are no quick and easy answers to the challenges facing rural senior centers. The great variability found in rural areas and populations requires center activities and approaches that are appropriate to local conditions and resources. The several examples presented in this chapter from across the nation show just how innovative rural center practitioners can be and often have to be.

Finally, this chapter has also reviewed briefly some of the basic research and policy questions that affect rural senior centers. There is much to be learned concerning the factors related to variations in rural center operation, programming, and participation patterns. Data are lacking on the relative effectiveness of different rural programming strategies, as are technical assistance and staff training materials on model service approaches. In addition, rural senior centers, like many community-based services, have developed and operated in a vaguely defined policy context. The roles best suited to and expected of senior centers have not been well formulated at the state and local levels. Who should rural senior centers be serving? What resources can or should be made available to rural centers, and where should they come from? What roles should senior centers play in *rural* community-based service systems? Answers to these questions will clarify the goals of rural senior centers, assist them in improving their effectiveness, and lead to a more comprehensive and better-coordinated rural community-based long-term care service system.

PART III

Resource Enhancement and Social Support

This section focuses on community-based services that, although clearly related to the health status and functioning of rural elders, are primarily aimed at enhancing their basic resources (in this case employment and housing) or ability to act as informal caregivers.

Chapter 6, by Dorfman and Ballantyne, begins with a thorough discussion of the need for rural elderly employment and training services—a need that is based in the lower incomes and higher poverty rates of this group and the out-migration of young adults from rural areas, which increases the importance of older persons as a source of labor and human capital. Dorfman and Ballantyne provide a succinct and thorough review of employment and job training programs and retirement services that are generally found in or have applicability to rural settings and present numerous examples of specific programs operating in rural areas. They also offer detailed discussion of the problems encountered in developing and providing employment and retirement services in rural settings. Some of the problems they identify include lack of rural resources, including money and trained staff; targeting of resources to frail older persons; lack of employment opportunities in rural areas; the urban orientation of most government programs; age discrimination in employment; lack of integrated service planning and provision; problems in accessing existing programs; and resistance of the rural elderly to participating in programs. Dorfman and Ballantyne also identify and discuss a number of responses to these problems. They end their chapter with a consideration of major research and policy issues related to the employment and retirement experiences and needs of rural elders. They argue for more advocacy for resources and for protection of existing government programs, such as social security and SSI, because rural elders tend to receive larger shares of their incomes from these sources than do nonrural elders. They note that geographic as well as inter-generational equity must be safeguarded in funding allocations and program targeting.

In Chapter 7, Prosper and Clark examine housing issues and programs affecting rural older persons. They begin by reminding the reader that the increased longevity of Americans, their desire to remain in their own dwellings as they age, and public policy trends that deemphasize institutional care have reinforced the importance of housing as a context in which age-related changes must be accommodated over many years. Prosper and Clark identify five areas that determine the degree to which housing can successfully support this "aging in place": affordability, safety and security, structural adaptability to accommodate physical and mental changes, availability of in-home supportive assistance, and easy access to personal care and health services. They present detailed statistics on the status of rural elderly housing, noting that the great majority of those living in rural elderly households are homeowners, but that they are more likely to be poor, to bear excessive housing costs, and to live in substandard dwellings than are their urban counterparts. In a detailed review, Prosper and Clark identify eight housing strategies that have proven successful in rural areas. They then discuss strategies for overcoming some of the barriers that can slow down the development and implementation of rural housing programs, including program, staff, and travel costs; lack of consumer access to the services; lack of program awareness among consumers, aging network practitioners, developers, and craftspersons; program inflexibility and bureaucratic red tape; lack of acceptance by the elderly; prohibitive zoning restrictions; affordability; and lack of knowledge of aging among housing professionals. Prosper and Clark conclude with a discussion of several research and policy issues related to housing programs for rural elders, such as ethical and liability issues for housing owners, service providers, and elderly tenants; defining the diverse housing needs and preferences of the many subgroups that make up the rural elderly; the need for practice-based models that illustrate how services can be successfully integrated with housing as an alternative to institution-based care; and, finally, the need for planning models that demonstrate successful rural community partnerships in meeting the care needs of older persons in housing environments.

The last chapter in Part III, by Schmall and Webb, addresses respite and adult day care. Respite care is designed primarily to provide temporary relief to informal caregivers (usually family members) from caregiving responsibilities and is provided in or outside of the home. Adult day care, on the other hand, provides relief to caregivers by bringing impaired older persons into a congregate setting that provides a range of services to the elders. Both respite and adult day services are generally much less likely to be found in rural than in urban areas, but can be successfully implemented in rural settings. Schmall and Webb begin with an overview of these services and an in-depth examination of the various approaches to providing them, with insights as to their applicability and problems in rural settings. Respite approaches they discuss include companion sitters, volunteer caregivers, and overnight respite. The adult day care approaches they review include those based at churches, at senior centers, at nursing homes, and at hospitals; portable adult day care; and adult day care homes. Schmall and Webb furnish a comprehensive discussion of the problems encountered in developing and providing these services in rural areas and offer strategies to overcome these difficulties. The problems include low rural population densities, transportation availability, and cost and a lack of linkages with both formal and informal support networks. Schmall and Webb point out that a large number of factors—such as lack of awareness and knowledge, apprehension, attitudes, timing, finances, reactions of the care recipient, and system inflexibility and bureaucracy—inhibit the use of these services even when they are available, and they provide useful insights on how to deal with these problems. Schmall and Webb end their chapter with a discussion of outstanding research and policy issues. They detail the many drawbacks of the existing research on these services as found in rural areas and characterize the data we do have as preliminary at best. They also ponder the implications of existing research for policy and practice issues and conclude that efforts to provide these services in rural areas must adopt a family-oriented approach, develop a strong and consistent funding base, give priority to in-home respite services, provide financial support to families, and reflect the realities and diversity of rural America.

6

Employment and Retirement
Services for the Rural Elderly

LORRAINE T. DORFMAN
ROBERT L. BALLANTYNE

Labor market problems encountered by some older workers and a lengthier retirement period for almost all workers are focusing attention on
the need for services related to employment, income maintenance, and
retirement. Such services have two major goals: to help individuals
maintain income adequacy in later life, and to promote overall quality
of life for older Americans. Employment and retirement services take
on particular significance in rural America because of the relative paucity of jobs in many rural areas, lower incomes than in urban areas, less
abundant and/or less accessible human services, and isolation from
large urban centers (Bird, 1990; Coward & Lee, 1985b; Hoppe, 1991;
Krout, 1986, 1991d; Nelson, 1980; Taietz & Milton, 1979).

This chapter describes existing employment and retirement services
for rural elderly, discusses problems encountered in developing and
providing those services and strategies that may overcome them, suggests programming directions for the future, and provides an overview
of research and policy issues relevant to service programming. We
conclude with a few brief summary comments.

The Need for Employment and Training Services

As some rural areas "depopulate" because of the migration of the
young to urban centers in search of better economic opportunities (Bird,

1990), older rural persons become an increasingly valuable source of human capital in many rural communities. It therefore makes sense to invest substantial resources in employment training and retraining services for middle-aged and older rural adults. Older rural adults can then fill existing jobs and any future jobs that may result from rural community development.

A fundamental reason for employment and training services, however, is that, on the average, the incomes of rural elders are significantly lower than those of their urban counterparts (Coward & Lee, 1985b; Kim, 1981; U.S. Bureau of the Census, 1987), reportedly approximately 20% lower (Krout & Dwyer, 1991). Government figures frequently use nonmetropolitan data (based on the population residing outside standard metropolitan statistical areas of 50,000 or more) to represent rural areas and small towns (Hoppe, 1991). In 1989, 15.3% of nonmetropolitan elderly aged 65 and above had incomes below the poverty level, whereas only 10.0% of metropolitan elderly in that age group had incomes below that level (U.S. Bureau of the Census, 1991a). Rural poverty among the elderly is the result of a complex set of factors, including low-paying jobs, sometimes considerable periods of unemployment, inadequate retirement benefits, and low public assistance (Watkins & Watkins, 1985). There is a significant regional impact in the incidence of rural poverty: the nonmetropolitan South has a far higher proportion of persons aged 65 and older living in poverty (20.9%) than does the nonmetropolitan West (9.7%), the Midwest (11.7%), or the Northeast (9.5%) (U.S. Bureau of the Census, 1991a).

The income status of older rural minorities and women is of particular concern. With respect to race, in 1989, 33.6% of nonmetropolitan black males aged 65 and older had incomes below the poverty level, compared with 19.0% of nonmetropolitan white males. Similar disparities were found in incomes of nonmetropolitan black and white females aged 65 and above (46.3% and 33.8% below poverty level, respectively). Among other large minority groups, in 1989, 26.9% of nonmetropolitan Hispanics aged 65 and older had incomes below the poverty level, compared with 13.3% of nonmetropolitan whites (U.S. Bureau of the Census, 1991a). With respect to gender, in 1989, 18.2% of nonmetropolitan females aged 65 and older had incomes below the poverty level, whereas only 11.2% of their male counterparts had incomes below that level (U.S. Bureau of the Census, 1991a). Taken together, these data indicate there is substantial racial/ethnic and gender variation in incomes of rural elderly.

It has been argued that rural areas do not have large or complex enough economic bases to provide enough jobs, and that federal employment programs are more available and spend more dollars in urban than in rural areas (Kim, 1981; Krout, 1986). Recent data indicate that nonmetropolitan labor force disadvantages continued to exist throughout the 1980s, with the nonmetropolitan underemployment rate (23.7%) continuing to exceed the metropolitan underemployment rate (15.2%) (Bird, 1990). (The underemployment rate combines the rates of adjusted unemployment and earnings below the individual poverty level.) Among mature adults aged 45-64, 3.9% of nonmetropolitan adults were unemployed, compared with 3.3% of their metropolitan counterparts (Bird, 1990). This nonmetropolitan disadvantage in employment did not hold after age 65, when most adults in both residential categories are retired. Mature nonmetropolitan dwellers aged 45-64 were also more likely to be working part-time or to have given up looking for jobs than were their metropolitan counterparts. The particularly unfavorable employment picture for nonmetropolitan women and minorities across age when compared with men and nonminorities was reflected in their relatively lower earnings as well as their higher rates of involuntary part-time employment and underemployment (Bird, 1990).

The Need for Retirement Services

Assistance in planning for retirement may be particularly important for rural elders because of their relatively lower incomes and the relatively higher incidence of self-employment in rural areas (11%) compared with urban areas (5%) (U.S. Bureau of the Census, 1983a). Self-employed elderly do not have the advantage of employer-sponsored retirement preparation programs to help in the transition to retirement; more important, they do not have company-funded pension plans to help finance their retirement. Self-employed rural adults may therefore require special help in financial planning. Recent data from a midwestern rural sample indicate that only a very small minority (3%) of rural elderly attend any kind of preretirement classes, seminars, or counseling sessions (Dorfman, 1989), compared with about 4%-5% of elders nationally (Atchley, 1991; Beck, 1984); this probably reflects the lower availability and accessibility of retirement planning programs in rural areas.

After retiring, the individual must find satisfying activities, such as recreational, educational, and volunteer activities, that can provide meaningful substitutes for the lost work role and that can help compensate for social losses that may accompany retirement. Generally, rural areas have fewer organizational resources to offer such activities than do urban areas (Krout, 1986, 1991d; Nelson, 1980; Taietz & Milton, 1979). This is particularly the case in very small villages and towns. A challenge, therefore, is to develop programs and services that will provide meaningful activities for retired rural elders within the resources of the rural community.

Approaches to Employment Services

Employment and Training Opportunities

Although private sector employment and training programs do exist, many of them on an ad hoc basis (Bureau of National Affairs, 1987), government programs provide a large share of employment and training programs for economically disadvantaged older persons. These programs may be particularly important for rural-dwelling older adults, who are generally more economically disadvantaged than are their urban counterparts. The major government programs are described below.

Title V of the Older Americans Act. The Older Americans Act (OAA) was first enacted in 1965. In 1973, OAA was amended to include Title V, which funded the Senior Community Service Employment Program (SCSEP). This program provides publicly subsidized minimum-wage jobs in community service positions in public and nonprofit organizational settings for persons aged 55 and older whose incomes are no more than 125% of poverty level (Hale, 1990). The goal is to place those older workers ultimately in unsubsidized employment.

SCSEP is administered by the U.S. Department of Labor. In many states the program is provided locally by Area Agencies on Aging (AAAs). In some states, several agencies administer the program, including community action agencies, the American Association of Retired Persons (AARP), and Green Thumb. Green Thumb is the major contractor for rural dollars (R. Freeman, personal communication, June 12, 1992). It is sponsored by the National Farmers Union with funds from the U.S. Department of Labor, and provides part-time employment in conservation, beautification, and community improvement projects in rural areas. Green Thumb is therefore a particularly useful source of employment for rural elderly (Atchley, 1991; Gelfand & Olsen, 1980).

A number of criticisms have been leveled at the traditional Title V model, including emphasis on income transfer and community service to the detriment of job placement, investment in specific types of job training, and incentives to work sites to outplace program participants (Sherman, Tirrillito, O'Rourke, & Nathanson, 1991). Title V, however, does accomplish the task for which it was intended—to provide income transfer to low-income seniors through tax-subsidized public service employment.

Job Training Partnership Act. The Job Training Partnership Act (JTPA) of 1982 is the latest in a series of comprehensive federal workforce development programs. The purpose of this legislation is to provide basic educational skills training and occupational skills training to "economically disadvantaged" and other persons with "multiple barriers to employment" in order to prepare them for employment and economic self-sufficiency (Bureau of National Affairs, 1987; Hale, 1990; Sandell, 1988). JTPA has several programs that provide employment and training activities to persons 55 years of age and older.

Title IIA is the largest part of the program. It aims to improve the employment situation of the most economically at-risk groups. As much as 10% of the population served under Title IIA does not have to be economically disadvantaged, but has to encounter other obstacles such as age and age discrimination (Hale, 1990). Title IIA provides assessment and testing, counseling, basic academic skills training, occupational skills training, job search training and assistance, and job placement.

Title IIA-3% is a special set-aside of Title IIA funding for persons 55 years of age or older. In general, the programs and activities are similar to all other Title IIA programs. It is significant to note that in terms of eligibility based upon income, the bulk of low-income seniors live just above the poverty guidelines, the eligibility threshold for JTPA. In some states, it is difficult to recruit enough persons to fill the 3% Older Workers Program.

Title III of JTPA provides monies for training, placement, and other related assistance to dislocated workers (Hale, 1990; Sandell, 1988). The program thus serves older adults who have lost jobs through plant closings or for other reasons.

Job Service. Job Service (also called the Employment Service or Employment Security) is another U.S. Department of Labor program. An important focus of this federal/state program is job placement. In order to deliver placement services, Job Service provides counseling, testing, referral, and a wealth of information and literature useful to job seekers.

Exemplary Employment Programming for Rural Application

Interagency caseload management. If public and nonprofit agencies have not already established close collaboration or coordinated operations in efforts to make programs more efficient and effective, current interest in reducing government spending might require it. What is needed are joint, integrated ventures among agencies providing services to rural persons who are age 55 or older. *Coordinated* or *single point of service* systems are delivery system designs for groups of agencies collaborating to blend services offered to particular populations.

Joint/integrated provision of service. All of the following are low-cost approaches to interagency cooperation and integration that are useful in employment and training services for older rural adults (Pennsylvania Department of Economic and Employment Development, 1989). *Joint outreach and recruitment* involves agency collaboration in providing public information to potential clients and sharing applicant information that would result in a specific constructive referral for service. *Universal application* is an interagency effort to reduce red tape for clients. In essence, agencies collaborate to create a single application and application process for a number of potential services. Then, through consultation with an interagency caseload management coordinator, clients receive "one-stop" service. This is particularly important in the rural environment, because travel is a considerable barrier to employment. *Interagency triage* is a method of interagency caseload reconciliation. Clients may work primarily with a single professional from a single agency, but that coordinator is meeting often with other agency personnel and, on a monthly basis, formally reading client dispositions into the mutual record and planning future services. *Cooperative follow-up/follow-along* and development and maintenance of a *peer/volunteer assistance network* are other important aspects of integrated interagency provision of services.

Employment and training conferences. These conferences are used to recruit, inform, and provide preliminary employment services to prospective rural clients. Additionally, workshops are given on such topics as skills and interests assessment, self-esteem/self-efficacy, and labor market orientation. In rural areas, telelink and video interactive conferences can be used to reach people in small towns and remote areas.

Job laboratory. A job laboratory is an interagency labor market orientation, career exploration, job search training resource room. Activities include employment assessment, career education, labor market orientation, résumé preparation, interview practice, and networking. The job laboratory is also a good resource for volunteer or peer assistance programs, where clients help other clients, with light to moderate professional support, to unrestricted access to training materials. The job laboratory can be taken on the road for delivery to rural persons at such sites as libraries or shopping centers. In our state, the East Central Iowa Employment and Training Consortium has offered a job laboratory as well as employment and training conferences for almost 10 years. Many other providers in the Midwest and elsewhere are now providing such services.

Entrepreneurial Activities

Some observers suggest that the economy of the United States in the twenty-first century may have more subsistence entrepreneurs and fewer persons supporting themselves with wages (e.g., Bergmann, 1983). Consequently, it is probably wise to develop employment programs for older rural adults that encourage more entrepreneurial activity (Robertson, 1985). There are a number of approaches that are currently being tried to encourage rural entrepreneurship and economic diversification.

Community college programs help people diversify their economic circumstances by developing open entry/open exit training programs to foster private enterprise and its diversification among rural citizens. For example, in Iowa, the Kirkwood Community College Rural Development Center has developed what it calls a "bottom-up" approach to spawning new small businesses, profitable small enterprises, cash crops, and alternatives to the wage economy in rural settings. The college holds workshops, business classes, business consultation, and specific training activities (Halder, 1991).

Extension service programs can be adapted to provide information to rural seniors about economic subsistence possibilities. The Kansas Center for Rural Initiatives at Kansas State University, for instance, provides services similar to those provided at the Kirkwood College program described above (Peak, 1990). Rural Alternatives, at Cornell University, is another economic diversification program that provides training and consultation to would-be entrepreneurs. Workshops, literature, and consultation are key elements of the program (Erikson, 1991).

SCORE (the Service Corps of Retired Executives) assists prospective and existing businesses with technical advice, and can be an important resource for entrepreneurial activity in rural areas.

Small business incubators are found at many universities and some community colleges. These facilities often offer space at reduced rent and access to academic consultation to emerging businesses. Additionally, business or research parks accommodate new business start-ups, joint ventures, and research. The Ben Craig Development Center at the University of North Carolina combines an incubator with a small business and technology center. The center supports individuals who have new business ideas by providing space, counseling, and shared secretarial support during the business start-up period (Halder, 1991).

Small business development centers, often affiliated with institutions of higher education, provide consultation to would-be entrepreneurs and to existing small businesses. Local governments and general-purpose business organizations may also maintain counseling services for new businesses. For example, the University of Iowa and the University of Northern Iowa have developed relationships with local governments and business organizations to facilitate long-term planning for rural development. Services include training and consultation for new business start-ups.

Crafts consignment networks provide marketing and support for homemade crafts. Senior centers or local stores often serve as outlets for these crafts. Many rural community action programs have experimented with crafts consignment programs as a means for seniors to produce goods and find a fair market. One such program began in Iowa in the early 1980s, where the Hawkeye Area Community Action Program provided retail outlets for handcrafted toys, utensils, and cloth goods. The shops took a retail markup. During the mid-1980s, the crafts network was spun off as a private venture. In Virginia, crafts made by the elderly are sold on consignment at an old general store operated by the Northern Neck-Middle Peninsula Area Agency on Agency. Senior centers throughout the 10-county planning and service area participate. This program receives funding from Title V, JTPA, and program income (Krout, 1990a).

Farmers' markets provide an opportunity for sale of locally grown agricultural products. Space can be provided in schools, churches, and parking lots of local businesses.

Approaches to Retirement and Recreation Services

The goal of retirement and recreation services is twofold: to facilitate adaptation of rural elders to retirement by providing assistance in planning for retirement, and to provide a social context for the continuation of meaningful and productive activities once retirement has occurred. A number of important services are discussed below.

Retirement Planning/Education

A central focus of retirement planning programs for rural adults should be financial planning and dissemination of financial information. Most retirement planning programs include assessment of major sources of income, such as social security, pensions, and investments, and of expected retirement expenditures. Increasingly, information on work after retirement is included. Rural retirement planning programs should help older rural adults find better ways to use the money they have by conserving resources and purchasing goods and services at the lowest possible cost (Harbert & Ginsberg, 1979). Programming should also include information on other issues that are particularly salient for rural elders, such as the move from farm to town and where and how to obtain health and human services.

Several subsets of rural elders may need particular help in retirement planning. Older rural widows, who may have had limited experience in handling finances, may be in special need of retirement planning and counseling. Minority elders, because of their relatively lower incomes, may also need special help in preparing for retirement. Farmers, who often say they expect to continue working but retire anyway, may be unprepared for retirement and may therefore require special assistance in retirement planning (Goudy, 1982).

Retirement preparation programs are often unavailable or inaccessible in rural areas. Use of sites such as churches, local businesses, and community centers may make it feasible, however, to offer programs in even very small villages and towns. In order to facilitate program delivery, rural service providers can develop retirement preparation programs in conjunction with the Cooperative Extension Service, community colleges, and senior centers. Rural service providers can also cooperate with local businesses in developing and delivering retirement preparation programs.

One example of a successful program is the AARP Women's Financial Counseling Program, which is designed to empower midlife and older women to make informed financial decisions. The program, consisting of six to eight weekly classes, is brought to local communities by nonprofit organizations such as the Cooperative Extension Service, senior centers, AAAs, and religious organizations, in cooperation with AARP. The program currently serves about 700 rural and urban communities in 48 states (American Association of Retired Persons, 1991b). In cooperation with the local chamber of commerce, a rural North Carolina AAA distributes a "retirement information package" that is mailed to potential in-migrants to the area. Information on housing, health services, and the like is included in the package (Krout, 1990a).

Recreational Programming

A first step for rural community planners and service providers is systematic collection of information on activities that retired and soon-to-be-retired rural people identify as meaningful. Recreational programming for retirement can then be planned and implemented in consultation with rural elders. It is important that recreational programming be designed to reflect the diverse recreational preferences of ethnic and racial minorities, of men and women, and of single and married persons within the particular rural community.

Organized recreational activities are frequently located in senior centers. In rural areas, however, lack of transportation may prevent access to these centers. One possibility is to offer decentralized recreational services, with just a few activities in small villages and towns, and a broader array of activities in larger rural communities (Krout, 1986). Recreational services in small towns and villages are likely to be offered in cooperation with church, civic, or fraternal organizations. Another way to increase recreational services in rural communities is to link rural recreational services to services in nearby urban communities. In New York State, senior citizens' clubs were organized in small villages and towns to meet regularly for social and recreational activities. These clubs then linked up with senior centers in larger communities for trips and other recreational events (Gelfand & Olsen, 1980). In Augusta, Georgia, an Area Agency on Aging has a contract with an urban-based theater to expand services to two rural communities. Services include courses in piano and voice training, dramatic reading, and facial expression and body movement. This cooperative effort provides opportunities for recreation as well as exposure to the arts (Krout, 1990a).

Volunteer Programs

Volunteering not only creates a "status-bearing, functional role" for the elderly (Salmon, 1979), it helps fill gaps in the formal service delivery system that exist in many rural communities. Many volunteer programs for the elderly are administered through ACTION, a federal agency. The Retired Seniors Volunteer Program (RSVP) provides volunteer opportunities for persons aged 60 and older in a variety of community settings, such as schools, libraries, hospitals, nursing homes, and day-care facilities. RSVP has agencies in more than 700 communities and is locally planned and sponsored (Gelfand & Olsen, 1980). The Foster Grandparents program provides low-income elderly with small stipends to work with children who have special needs. The Senior Companion Program also provides small stipends for low-income elderly to work with special needs elderly in their own homes or in adult day care, nursing homes, or hospitals (Gelfand & Olsen, 1980).

In addition to these federally sponsored programs, rural communities currently organize many volunteer activities to fit their specific needs through local senior centers, churches, schools, and civic organizations. An intergenerational "buddy system" in rural Pennsylvania brings together elders and elementary and high school students. Participants meet a few times a month for joint recreational activities or just to visit. Volunteers in a rural Michigan county deliver talking and large-print books to homebound elderly throughout the county. The program is based in and coordinated by the local library (Krout, 1990a).

Continuing Education

Educational programs for older rural persons are often limited; however, a number of agencies are currently offering continuing education programs for both retired and preretired rural adults. Community colleges, who have continuing education as part of their mandate, offer many noncredit courses either at the colleges themselves or through community education classes in outlying communities. The Cooperative Extension Service, local YMCAs, and senior centers also offer continuing education classes, often in cooperation with community colleges. Recent advances in telecommunications now bring continuing education programs to residents of many small communities and to the open countryside.

One continuing education program is called Elderhostel; it provides short-term educational programs to persons aged 60 and older at colleges and universities throughout the United States (Atchley, 1991; Gelfand & Olsen, 1980). This program might be of interest to rural elders who are able to travel to the institutions of their choice for short stays of a week or two. An education program in rural South Dakota, called DARE, was developed cooperatively by a community college and a senior center. This program, which includes a wide variety of courses, ranging from creative writing to health, was first offered at a senior center and later expanded to rural satellite centers in communities of fewer than 500 population. The program uses special educational materials provided by the National Council on Aging and the National Endowment for the Humanities (Price, 1980).

Strategies for Overcoming Problems Encountered in Developing and Providing Services

Adequate financing of employment and retirement services is of fundamental concern. The larger proportion of elderly and the more limited tax base of rural compared with urban communities result in higher demand placed on limited resources for social services (Nelson, 1980). There is currently a strong trend toward putting resources into services for the frail elderly. Although such services are important, there is also a need to put resources into services for well elderly, especially programs that will help maintain income and promote overall quality of life. Practitioners must be strong advocates in particular for existing employment and training programs, and for increased funding for new and existing programs.

A particular problem in rural areas is lack of fit between government employment programs and rural economies that do not afford abundant employment options. Existing legislation is substantially tailored to meet urban needs, with employment programs less fitted to addressing rural problems such as lack of transportation, lack of a wage economy, and lack of local economic diversity. We cannot expect to see the same kind of results from rural employment and training programs as from urban programs, because rural areas have smaller labor markets to absorb job seekers. Entrepreneurial or diversification alternatives are necessary.

In addition, age discrimination in employment is a real phenomenon, despite legislation to the contrary (the Age Discrimination in Employment Act). Becoming informed about individual civil rights and the law can be helpful for would-be job seekers. The Civil Rights Commissions and the Equal Employment Opportunity Commission can help with particular problems, as can legal assistance organizations.

In provision of services, lack of truly integrated planning and provision of services among agencies with overlapping interests is a particular concern in many rural areas. Because services are often widely dispersed, planners and program specialists need to be especially committed to fostering interorganizational cooperation (Nelson, 1980). For one thing, cooperative assessments should be undertaken to determine the need for specific services. Coordinated outreach should also be undertaken to increase rural elders' awareness of employment and retirement services. Finally, sharing of resources, interagency planning, and joint evaluation of services are all important for adequate service provision.

It is commonplace for agencies in rural areas to have much smaller professional staffs than do urban agencies. Rural practitioners are therefore more likely than their urban counterparts to be generalists (Ginsberg, 1976; Watkins & Watkins, 1985). In addition, relatively more staff time in rural areas must be spent on indirect services, such as administration and coordination, than on direct services (Nelson, 1980). An important resource for supplementing professional staff in rural communities is use of trained volunteers and peers.

Access to employment and retirement services is another major problem in many rural communities. A number of strategies can be utilized to transport older people to these services. Volunteer transportation can be organized if no public transportation is available. Practitioners need to recruit volunteer drivers and coordinate schedules to match drivers with the needs of older clients (Harbert & Ginsberg, 1979). Vehicles belonging to schools, churches, and other organizations can be utilized to provide transportation to rural elders during off-peak hours. Another strategy is to bring employment and retirement services directly to rural elders by means of mobile delivery services and by rotation of service providers.

Finally, a subtler problem in utilization of employment and retirement services is resistance of the rural elderly themselves. Values of individualism and self-reliance have traditionally been considered more important to rural than to nonrural people (Krout, 1986; Melton &

Childs, 1983). Rural elderly may therefore have negative attitudes about accepting government assistance. They may also feel hesitant about accepting retraining opportunities for jobs, both prior to and after retirement. Additionally, some may be fearful of employment and retirement preparation programs because of low self-esteem or self-efficacy. Trained counselors who are sensitive to the values and needs of rural elders can help reduce these problems in the underutilization of programs.

Needs and Programming Directions for the Future

A number of directions are critical for future employment and retirement programming. The suggestions that follow are not prioritized; all can be expected to achieve positive results.

More job training and placement services are needed for older rural adults in order to combat skills obsolescence in a changing job market. Successful older worker programs include adequate assessment of participants' skills, abilities, and interests; occupational skills training; staff knowledge of participants' employment potential and the local labor market; job search training; job match; and coordination with other programs and agencies (Sandell & Baldwin, 1990).

Cooperation with the private sector is important in this context. Additionally, efforts should be made to increase placements in existing government programs such as Green Thumb and Senior Community Service Employment Programs. Information about employment opportunities should be disseminated widely, possibly through publication of an employment directory or newsletter. A toll-free "warm line" could also disseminate information about employment opportunities.

More financial counseling programs are needed. Older rural women and minorities, along with the underemployed and unemployed, are in particular need of such services. Itinerant financial counselors and retirement planners can be brought in to visit rural areas on a rotating basis. Additionally, rural adults who reside in the community can be trained as peer educators to provide financial counseling.

Rural community development is needed to help create jobs. Some rural development specialists advocate attracting older migrants to stimulate local economies; however, the number of such migrants is relatively small (Hoppe, 1991). Combined with a large indigenous rural elderly population, however, retired migrants can stimulate expansion of the recreational and health sectors. Tourism is an additional direction for rural community development.

Future employment and retirement programming should include more direct involvement of employers. Efforts should be made to educate local employers, possibly in the form of seminars, about the capacities of older workers, and encouragement given to provide more part-time employment for older workers. More on-site employment training should be offered. Furthermore, encouragement of employers to adopt retirement planning programs can result in such payoffs as improved morale, public relations, and possibly earlier retirement of workers.

Programs should be introduced to recruit and train volunteers as job counselors and peer educators to help combat problems created by an insufficient professional labor pool. Fitchen (1990) suggests that older in-migrants to rural communities are a valuable resource for volunteer activities. Volunteering will not only reduce the possibility of migrants' isolation, but, along with the volunteer efforts of "old-timers," will contribute to the well-being of their communities. It is very important for service providers to coordinate the work of such informal helpers and to integrate their activities into the formal delivery system.

Finally, future programming should make greater use of modern telecommunications to inform large audiences of rural adults about employment and retirement services, and to provide educational programming. Written materials such as newsletters are also valuable for supplementing television, video, and radio presentations.

Research and Policy Issues

Research Needs

A great deal more empirically based information is necessary if we are to have adequate information on which to base future employment and retirement services. Specific research needs include the following:

1. Comparative studies are needed to determine the degree to which work and retirement differ in rural and nonrural locations (e.g., the amount and nature of employment, work after retirement, factors related to retirement adjustment). Programs and services can then be designed that are unique to the rural environment and that are not based on the dominant urban model.

2. Research on the need for and current and potential contributions of older rural workers is essential. Such research is particularly important in light of the "depopulation" of some rural areas caused by the out-migration of the young to urban areas in search of better economic opportunities.

3. More research is needed on variations in work and retirement among rural communities. Multisite local and regional studies will yield information that can be used to develop employment and retirement programs that are appropriate for specific local populations.

4. More information is needed on variations in employment and retirement by gender, race, socioeconomic status, and marital status, and how these factors interact with residential location.

5. More research is needed on rural service utilization, including examination of how attitudinal, behavioral, and environmental factors interact to affect service utilization among different groups of rural elderly.

6. Longitudinal research is called for to provide information on how the need for employment and retirement services changes over time. Panel studies can assess not only age-related changes, but also how the need for services changes prior to and after retirement.

7. More investigations of the impact of entrepreneurial activity on rural elders are needed. Likewise, a stronger academic picture of the "underground" economies at work in rural settings—a microeconomic analysis—will be necessary for service planning to be effective. Most of the statistics currently amassed by the Bureau of Labor Statistics measure broad macroeconomic trends.

8. Evaluation studies are imperative to assess the relationship between employment and retirement services and outcomes. Both immediate program evaluations and longer-term follow-ups should be undertaken to provide information that can be used to modify existing programs and to implement new ones.

Policy Issues

Several policy issues are central for future employment and retirement programming in rural areas. First, advocacy is needed in order to maintain and increase support for rural employment and training programs. An important policy issue in this context is intergenerational equity: Policies and programs must come to grips with and attempt to balance the employment and training needs of both older and younger rural persons.

Advocacy is also needed to help protect direct income supports such as social security, Medicare, and SSI, and for health and human services. Rural practitioners and community leaders must be strong advocates for all of these programs. Advocates for the rural elderly must also work to ensure that this subpopulation receives its fair share of government-funded programs and services. Changes in legislation regarding transfer payments must be closely monitored, because rural elderly receive a larger share of their income from these payments than do urban elderly (Hoppe, 1991).

Setting priorities in the above areas is of great importance. For instance, is it more beneficial to emphasize job training and retraining programs or improvement of direct income supports for older rural adults? Likewise, deciding who should bear primary financial responsibility for services is of major importance. Should financial responsibility be borne primarily by federal, state, or local governments, or by a combination or joint effort of these agencies? Or should the private sector play a larger role in the financing of services, possibly in cooperation with the public sector?

Training and recruitment of rural service professionals is another policy issue that must be addressed. Resources need to be put into educating professionals in rural gerontology as well as in specific content areas such as finances and recreation (Kim, 1981). It is important not only to train and recruit professionals for the rural labor pool, but also to do more outreach and continuing education for practitioners who are already in the field, in order to update and improve their skills.

Summary and Conclusions

In this chapter we have examined a number of existing and alternative approaches to employment and retirement services for older rural adults and identified a number of problems in the development and provision of such services. Major problems include financing, access, staffing, and integration of services. We have proposed a number of directions for future programming of employment and retirement services: more and improved job training and placement services, more financial counseling, greater involvement of employers, more intensive recruitment and training of rural service professionals, greater use of peer educators and volunteers, and use of modern telecommunications.

It is important to point out that older rural Americans' employment is impeded not only by job loss and lack of job search, job training and retraining, and job placement services, but also by such factors as poor economic conditions, age discrimination, and poor health (Sandell, 1988). The policy solutions to employment difficulties therefore require a broad societal commitment to improved economic and social conditions as well as to providing services that will ameliorate existing employment problems. Similarly, a broad societal commitment to improved economic and social conditions, as well as to retirement-specific services, is needed to reduce problems that may be associated with retirement. Such preventive and ameliorative efforts would help to improve the overall quality of life of older rural Americans.

7

Housing America's Rural Elderly

VERA PROSPER
STOCKTON CLARK

The primary housing-related preference of older people is to "age in place" (American Association of Retired Persons, 1990; Prosper, 1990b). However, increasing longevity has resulted in growing numbers of individuals surviving lengthier periods with the chronic mental and physical frailties commonly seen in old-old age. According to 1992 data from the Research Unit of the New York State Office for the Aging, the need for some assistance to continue living viably in a housing environment rises from approximately 15% among those aged 65-69 to 51% among those aged 85 and over. Thus, although the elderly prefer to live out their later years in their own homes, five major housing-related needs compromise their ability to make aging in place a workable choice: affordability, safety and security, structural adaptability to accommodate physical and mental changes, availability of in-home supportive assistance, and easy access to personal care and health services.

Public policy trends in health and aging support older people's preference to age in place by deemphasizing institutional care and promoting the development of a continuum of in-home and community-based services as a strategy for containing the rising costs of long-term care. However, there has been little collaboration among health and aging networks and the housing industry in planning and coordinating the integration of housing and services. Until very recently, the major public response to elderly housing needs was aimed at affordability. Federal and state housing agencies concentrated on developing affordable units and giving financial aid for rent and home repair. Public programs to develop housing/services models or to incorporate special design features have been minimal; issues of housekeeping, meals, personal care, emotional and cognitive impairments, chronic disability, and the like have been considered discrete responsibilities of the aging and health networks. However, as these public policy and demographic trends continue, the elderly increasingly rely on the size, environmental aspects, location, and condition of their homes to provide the viable foundation for meeting their increasingly complex daily living needs. The function of "housing" has evolved beyond simply ensuring basic shelter to providing a living environment that will accommodate aging-related changes over the long term.

This chapter describes the efforts of public and private groups to create such viable living environments for rural older persons. As used here, the term *rural* refers to geographic areas of the country defined by the U.S. Bureau of the Census as "nonmetropolitan." The housing status of rural elderly and policy issues related to housing these older persons are discussed. The greatest portion of the chapter is devoted to describing eight housing strategies that have proven successful in rural areas in addressing the five major housing need areas identified above. Each strategy is defined, the benefits for rural elderly are described, barriers to development are identified, and means for overcoming these barriers are suggested.

Rural Elderly Housing Status

In 1989, there were 20.1 million households in the United States headed by persons 65 years or older (U.S. Bureau of the Census, 1991b). Of these, 27% (5.4 million) were in the rural areas of the country. Of the rural elders living in these households, 80% are homeowners (Belden, 1992), with 70% having paid-off mortgages (Lazere et al., 1989). In 1985, 27% of rural elderly households (1.5 million) were poor; that is, they had incomes below the federal poverty rate of $5,156/$6,503 (compared with 19% of nonrural elderly), and 61% had incomes below 200% of poverty (Lazere et al., 1989). Some 31% of rural elderly householders spent 30% or more of their income on housing costs (Lazere et al., 1989). Given that the great majority of the mortgages of these householders are paid off, excessive housing costs represent the rising costs of utilities, property taxes, insurance, maintenance, and repair. Two-thirds of poor rural elderly householders are individuals living alone, the majority of them women (Lazere et al., 1989). A total of 13% of rural elderly householders occupy substandard housing, compared with 9% of metropolitan elderly householders. Thus rural elderly represent 27% of total elderly households, but 43% of total elderly substandard households and 57% of severely substandard elderly households (Lazere et al., 1989).

Despite some overall similarities, the elderly are the most diverse of all age groups. The needs and preferences of subsegments of this population vary significantly. A rural/urban taxonomy is helpful in defining needs and developing appropriate housing strategies because the environmental and economic characteristics of a community vary according to geographic location, and these distinctions have a direct impact on an elderly population's circumstances. For example, urban elderly are primarily renters. Because rural elderly are predominantly homeowners, their risk of physical isolation during the frail years is increased. The natural support and informal oversight systems that often develop among older renters because of proximity in a housing project are not available among scattered rural homesites. The risk of isolation is exacerbated where increasingly restrictive land-use regulations limit the informal support opportunities traditionally available by adding extensions or trailers to rural homesites to accommodate extended family members or returning grown children. Also, for homeowners, responsibility for upkeep and repair remains with the individual even when agility and health diminish. However, unlike renters, older homeowners have home equity that can represent a sizable and potentially usable financial asset.

In addition to geographic differences, because "old age" spans a range of more than 40 years, income status, functional profiles, family and cultural status, and preferences of older people vary dramatically among elderly age cohorts. Therefore, a variety of housing options and programs are necessary to respond appropriately to the diversity that characterizes this population's subgroups.

Successful Housing Strategies
for Rural Older Persons

The options described below have proven successful in rural communities across the United States. They promote viable aging in place by addressing the five major areas of housing-related needs of rural older persons: affordability, safety, accommodating design, supportive assistance, and access to health care.

One-Stop-Shop Housing Counseling

One-stop-shop housing counseling is a recent development in response to the multiple housing-related problems encountered as more frail elderly continue living in the community. It is a housing case management service in which a counselor assesses an older person's housing circumstances and needs, inventories all available housing-related resources, and coordinates the delivery of these services, including finding alternative housing and assistance in relocating. The counselor also refers clients to other agencies for non-housing-related services and financial assistance. Housing counseling programs are operated by community voluntary agencies, are generally free to elderly clients, and are funded by a variety of public and private sources such as state and local governments, legislative and foundation grants, and local and in-kind contributions.

Benefits

The elderly are typically unfamiliar with available community services. In addition, rural elderly are far from services and lack transportation to get to them. Rural older people are receptive to one-stop-shop counseling programs because counselors exhibit sensitivity regarding the personal traits of the elderly—they make home visits, present services in a nonthreatening way, customize service plans to the unique needs and preferences of individuals, and involve older persons in self-directed decision making. A further advantage of this type of service is that it requires an elderly person to interact with only a single counselor for comprehensive assessment and service planning. These features reduce or eliminate the psychological barriers rural elderly often experience: mistrust of government, intimidation by complex public programs operated by different departments and requiring differing applications, and the loss of self-respect and self-reliance felt when applying for public assistance.

Barriers and Strategies

The main barrier to development of one-stop-shop counseling is its cost. Housing case management is staff-intensive and, in rural areas, travel-intensive. Program administrative costs are typically not shared by the community services accessed on behalf of the older homeowner. There also continues to be disagreement about which network should assume responsibility (and cost) for providing housing counseling. It is seen as a "soft service" by housing agencies that measure output in bricks and mortar. It is unfamiliar territory to aging network providers who target such personal services as meals, personal care, and psychological counseling. When public funds are tight, housing counseling programs are generally the first to be cut because they are neither bricks and mortar nor basic necessities such as food or health care.

Funding agencies often prioritize the allocation of scarce monies to programs showing high numbers of tangible outcome units. Stable funding for housing counseling can be better assured by making this service part of a larger program that includes financial counseling for families, home equity conversion counseling, home-sharing programs, home repair programs, and so on. Housing counseling efforts can also be meshed with the wider service network to integrate housing assessments into traditional health/social case management services.

Home Repair Programs

Home repair programs range from minor fix-it programs that include such jobs as fixing toilets, caulking windows, replacing locks, snaking water lines, patching holes, and minor electrical work to moderate rehabilitation programs that include the replacement of the major systems of the home: heating, plumbing, electrical, sewer, and structural work. Many home repair programs are targeted specifically to elderly homeowners. The goals behind all these programs are to maintain the community's housing stock at a standard level and to assist persons who are physically or financially unable to maintain their own homes.

The two major federally sponsored home repair programs are the Farmers Home Administration Section 504 Program, which provides grants and loans to low-income elderly homeowners, and the U.S. Department of Energy's Weatherization Program, which contracts with voluntary agencies to provide outreach and energy-saving home improvements at no charge to low-income families. The federal Home Energy Assistance Program (HEAP) is not a repair program, but provides financial aid to low-income families to pay heating bills. To fill the continuing gap in demand, states' housing and aging agencies have developed a variety of grant and loan home repair and moderate rehabilitation programs that piggyback the federal programs. A large variety of community-based home repair programs are in place across the country that have been developed and are operated by community groups and funded by local businesses and governments, legislative grants, and creative fund-raising efforts. In addition, localities devote HUD's Community Development Block Grant monies and Home Program dollars to home repair services, channeling funds through churches, housing agencies, and other voluntary groups.

Benefits

According to the American Association of Retired Persons (1991a), 40% of rural elderly householders live in housing stock that was built prior to 1950. Many of these homes are uninsulated, lack modern features, and have not received major overhauls in plumbing, electrical, or heating systems since being built. When faced with choices in spending insufficient income, older persons will typically forgo regular home maintenance and repair to pay for food, medicine, medical care, and heat. Home repair programs help elderly people age in place by increasing the safety, security, and comfort of their homes, and by reducing the operating costs of homeownership.

Repair programs constitute a very cost-effective strategy for helping older people age in place. For example, New York State's emergency repair program for the elderly (RESTORE) rehabilitated 723 homes in its first two years, at an average cost of $2,371 per household (Prosper, 1991). For a modest infusion of money, often augmented by family and community efforts, the fiber of the rural community is reinforced at the same time the condition and value of the housing stock is maintained.

Barriers and Strategies

Barriers to rural home repair programs include insufficient funds, consumer lack of access to the service, and program inflexibility. Federal, state, or local program funds rarely meet the repair needs of rural elderly homeowners, and required regulatory paperwork often impinges on timely service delivery. Thus repairs are often delayed or postponed indefinitely, leaving residents living in dangerous and unhealthy conditions. The large distances that separate homes in rural America make it particularly difficult and costly for providers to identify needy elderly families and to deliver repair services in cost-efficient ways. Also, individual programs often target specific needs, such as energy-related or small repairs, or programs will cap the dollars allotted per home, leaving single programs unable to correct the multiple problems found in many older persons' homes.

To address these barriers, states and localities have dedicated blocks of funds for innovative "emergency" repair programs, with guidelines that mandate immediate repairs in situations that pose an imminent threat to the older resident's health or safety. Others have instituted "packaging," a case management approach to assessing and delivering home repair and energy-saving services. The packager coordinates delivery of all applicable housing-related services available, thus maximizing benefits to each household.

Local programs have been successful in maintaining long-term funding by creatively joining forces with other community networks to address the needs of several populations. Some examples include forming partnerships with a local school's work-study program for students to learn home repair skills, using retired skilled craftspersons as mentors to young employees as an intergenerational initiative, providing cosponsorship and public relations publicity for local businesses in exchange for free or at-cost materials, negotiating agreements with local businesses to receive "throwaway" materials, and using community and school volunteer and sweat equity efforts in concert with public monies to maximize available repair benefits.

Home Equity Conversion

Home equity conversion (HEC) programs convert the equity in an elderly person's home into cash payments that are repaid only when that resident moves from the home or title to the home changes. Payments can be lump sums or monthly payments and are considered loans against the home. Future repayment includes the principal loaned, accumulated compounded interest, mortgage recording fees and taxes, and any additional charges such as insurance, underwriting, and processing fees. A variety of HEC models are available, including the more traditional ones such as sale/leaseback arrangements, life estates, and property tax deferral, as well as innovative instruments such as the line of credit and various reverse mortgage plans. Their varying features make each model an attractive option to a particular segment of older people, depending upon their age, health status, income, value of the home, and perceived need for the money. The features of any one HEC program make it workable for elderly with a certain configuration of characteristics. For example, a 10-year loan may be inappropriate for a healthy 65-year-old, but may be very helpful for an 85-year-old needing extensive nursing care.

Benefits

The benefit of HEC is its capacity to unlock the buying power of a valuable fixed asset at a time in life when income has dramatically decreased. It is workable because repayment is deferred. HEC promotes aging in place by adding income to help pay for daily living expenses, housing costs, transportation, health care services, and supportive assistance. When elderly persons can use their own funds for these expenses, their self-esteem and continued independence are enhanced because they feel less reliant upon public benefits and worry less about becoming a burden to other family members.

Barriers and Strategies

An objection to HEC by some elderly is the accumulated interest cost on the loans. Others are reluctant to incur debt or find it emotionally impossible to put a lien on the home they have worked a lifetime trying to own. Others wish to leave their homes to their children. Further, for homes with low asset values, the accumulated HEC costs over a long period may not allow high enough monthly payments to warrant investment in the program.

Because HEC is a solution that is costly and ultimately results in the loss of the home, it should not be considered in isolation but, rather, as one option among many that can solve housing or service needs. Generally, community counseling and service organizations are trained about HEC programs and include them in their menu of alternative housing assistance programs.

Lending institutions are often reluctant to offer HEC plans because the long-term nature of these loans involves a potential financial risk for them. Some offer only limited-term instruments (generally 10 years) to minimize this risk. Lenders often feel a public relations skittishness about short-term HEC plans as the potential exists that a loan repayment will come due, forcing an elderly resident's loss of the home and unwanted relocation. Thus lenders typically engage community agencies to provide a counseling component to HEC programs as a means of addressing consumer protection and public relations issues. The federal Department of Housing and Urban Development's National HEC Mortgage Insurance Program addresses lender concerns by underwriting, through the Federal National Mortgage Association (Fannie Mae), a variety of HEC models and by mandating consumer counseling by an impartial community agency. Private companies are also emerging across the country that provide HEC loans. Some states have developed state HEC counseling programs to educate elderly consumers about this option as an alternative housing-related program. States could make HEC more viable for rural owners of low asset value homes by subsidizing the administrative fees and interest charges through a public revolving loan fund.

Accommodating Design

In the past 10 years, rapid advances have been made in technological and architectural design developments to create adaptable, universal housing. Design examples include height-adjustable sinks and counters, single-lever faucets, task lighting, bathtub and elevator seats, thresholds flush with the floor, contrasting colors for walls/floors, acoustic features to eliminate background noises, no nosings on stairs, frost-free refrigerators, large-room listening devices, anthropomorphic furniture design, computerized home command centers, comprehensible interior layouts, and building design to enhance interior/exterior orientation. Such design features compensate for impairments and frailties by not requiring the levels of strength, stamina, agility, vision, hearing, and cognition typical of younger persons. Many of these features add little (about 1%) or no extra cost if incorporated during the initial construction phase or during planned rehabilitation of existing structures (Koncelik, 1982).

As the benefits of adaptable, universal housing have become more widely acknowledged as a way to enhance the continued self-management and independence of frail elderly persons, as well as younger persons with disabilities, public and private groups are promoting its use through regulatory changes and research and educational initiatives. For example, North Carolina, New York, and Florida have developed easy-reference adaptable design manuals. New York State's aging and housing agencies have collaborated to include aging-specific design guidelines in the state's manual for capital-funding applicants. HUD's revised Section 202 regulations include funding eligibility for aging-accommodating design features. Gerontologists, architects, design researchers, and academics have published articles, books, and manuals on this subject. Private organizations have developed various versions of the National Association of Home Builders' Smart House concept, a programmable integrated home wiring system that carries power, audio, video, and data transmission signals that communicate electronically with all electric and electronic devices and appliances in the home. Several organizations, such as the Travelers Company, have constructed model homes for public display that demonstrate the adaptable, universal housing concept.

Benefits

Adaptable housing accommodates the physical and mental changes that can occur during the aging process. An accommodating environment extends an older person's capacity for self-management and independence, reduces reliance on others for daily activities, delays or avoids institutionalization and, thus, enhances competence, self-esteem, and privacy in the later years (Prosper, 1990a).

Barriers and Strategies

Barriers to the use of adaptable design features in rural areas have included developers', craftspersons', and consumers' lack of awareness of the concept and its benefits; lack of knowledge about where to buy items such as adjustable sinks or room listening devices; and cost parameters for public housing that limit the use of many special features.

Much of the effort to counter these barriers has occurred at the state government level or through research and academic organizations. States have developed and disseminated technical assistance manuals, and a variety of private and public organizations have conducted conferences and workshops that have proven successful in educating professionals about the relationship between aging and the environment, the impact of adaptable design, and where to purchase specific items. Local voluntary groups and aging advocates can play a larger role in these efforts by enlisting joint sponsorship of local businesses, builders' associations, and banks to target education sessions to local developers, planning and zoning officials, legislators, and service providers. Much of the technical expertise and many of the printed materials needed for such workshops are available at low or no cost.

Community groups can also use new opportunities offered by recent regulatory changes to educate planners about the design of community-based senior housing. For example, to access capital funds under the National Affordable Housing Act, HUD requires state and local jurisdictions to submit a comprehensive housing plan that has been subject to public hearings, review, and comment. In addition, some jurisdictions include an advisory body of community groups to assist in fashioning the housing plan. HUD's revised Section 202 Program requires that funding applications include an aging services plan that has been certified by the Area Agency on Aging. This is an opportunity for aging service providers to work closely with developers in the initial design stages of senior housing development.

Secondary Units (Elder Cottages and Accessory Apartments)

Elder cottages (also known as ECHO housing, PLUS units, and granny flats) are small, freestanding units that are factory built with the same material, design, and construction standards as a traditional single-family home. Each contains a kitchen, bedroom, living/dining area, bathroom, and storage spaces. In long-standing traditional use, an elder cottage is temporarily sited in the backyard of a son's or daughter's home for use by a frail elderly parent. However, as current housing costs have escalated, developers are creating elder cottage cluster developments for rent or sale to older persons, or to mixed ages as affordable intergenerational housing. A community building can be added to the cluster, and linkages can be established with community service agencies for coordinated delivery of social, supportive, and health services.

An accessory apartment (commonly known as a mother-in-law apartment) is a private unit within an existing single-family home and contains a kitchen, bathroom, bedroom, living area, storage spaces, and separate egress to the outside. It is created by converting a garage, attic, basement, or bedrooms of the present home, or can be a new addition. An apartment can be created in a son's or daughter's home for use by a frail elderly parent, or an elderly person's home can be adapted to include such an apartment, with the older person choosing to live in either section and renting out the other.

Benefits

Secondary units provide the emotional security of having someone nearby (particularly the family's supportive assistance), the reduced upkeep burdens of a smaller home, use of personal green space for gardening and sitting, affordability, the convenience of proximity for caregiver families, and maximized privacy at a time in life when frailty compromises independent living. High construction standards, high re-sale value, and the ability to be re-sited without damage make elder cottages a good investment for reusable housing stock.

Barriers and Strategies

Although older people find secondary units to be attractive options, many factors inhibit their widespread use. Prohibitive zoning language is the major barrier. Critics equate elder cottages with trailers, or feel that second structures will change the character of a residential street. Some think the community's infrastructure will be strained, or that the units' future rental uses cannot be controlled. Community workshops targeted to zoning and planning officials, key community leaders, and service providers have proven successful in educating people about these housing options and in alleviating critics' fears. Workshops use land-use professionals, gerontologists, and unit manufacturers to demonstrate how secondary units can fit into a community's master plan for meeting comprehensive housing needs. Training is also provided on how to fashion zoning language effectively to define the parameters for the units' uses and the conditions governing their removal or reuse. Model zoning ordinances have been developed by communities across the United States and by the American Association of Retired Persons.

As most older people prefer to not move, secondary units are generally chosen when frailty demands it. However, even when an older person would choose this option, families may not have sufficient yard room to site a cottage or house space to include an apartment. Many elderly have no available family, or have children who are themselves elderly, or do not choose to move to distant locations where family members live. Some elderly and their families do not wish to live close together. When frail, some elderly cannot take on the burdens of adapting their own homes to include accessory apartments or the burdens of renting their own homes. Elder cottage clusters address many of these issues.

Public funding programs have been developed to promote the use of secondary units. Fannie Mae's Senior Housing Options Program underwrites conventional mortgages for either option. Elder cottage clusters are eligible for capital funding from the Farmers Home Administration and the Department of Housing and Urban Development. Some states provide grants/loans to community groups and municipalities to develop both options for rent or sale to low-income older persons. An elder cottage rental program addresses local concerns such as timely removal of vacant units and control of rental practices. A public development grant program, with very low rental charges, could provide a workable option in poorer rural areas of the country where the $35,000 purchase/siting cost of a cottage is still unaffordable.

Home Sharing (Match-Up Programs and Shared Living Residences)

Match-Up home-sharing programs for the elderly are a new, formalized version of an age-old idea. These programs bring together individuals seeking affordable housing with homeowners who have room to spare. Match-Up programs differ from commercial home matching services in that an older person is part of each match; extensive compatibility screening is part of the process; sharers are assisted in drawing up sharing agreements; and program staff stay involved to assist sharers in resolving conflicts, dissolving matches, rematching or seeking alternative arrangements, and linking with needed community services.

Particulars are determined by the sharers, and can range from equally shared financial and upkeep burdens of running the home, to purely rental arrangements, to arrangements involving reduced rent or rent-free housing in exchange for social companionship or services such as yard work, housekeeping, and transportation. Successful matches may be short- or long-term. They can involve two older persons or can be an intergenerational match that includes an older person and a college student, health care staff person, single parent, younger couple, disabled younger person, or other nonelder.

In a shared living residence, 3 to 10 unrelated persons live together as a family in a large home or apartment that is owned or leased by a community agency. Residents have private bedrooms and share bathrooms, living areas, kitchen, and yard. They pay rent and share homemaking tasks and companionship. Resident groups can be all elderly or an intergenerational mix. A residence can include a staff person who provides housekeeping and meal services, facilitates problem solving, and assists residents in linking with community services.

Both types of home-sharing programs are operated by voluntary and public agencies, with public funding or grant support; there is typically no fee charged to sharers for the matching service.

Benefits

Sharing is a good rural option because of the number of aging persons living alone in large family homes or in isolated open areas. These options can delay costly institutionalization and allow older persons to remain in their own homes or communities at a time when independence is compromised by a need for financial aid, supportive assistance, companionship, or simply the presence of another person in the home. Sharing makes more efficient use of rural housing stock. Intergenerational models that include oversight by community agencies provide an affordable housing option for single parents and young adults who cannot meet their daily living expenses from the low-paying service sector jobs that are typical in many rural areas.

Barriers and Strategies

Privacy is extremely important to older people. Many elders will choose a shared residence arrangement only when aging-related impairments preclude private living. Thus those in a shared residence group may be too frail to live without assistance. Successful models include staff who live on- or off-site and who assist with homemaking, coordination of activities, conflict resolution, and linkage to community services. Other successful models are intergenerational, linking younger persons' needs for affordable rent and older residents' needs for the assistance provided by younger residents.

Restrictive zoning language can be a barrier, although recent court decisions have been helpful through favorable definition of what constitutes a family. Because sharing is a low preference among the elderly, it may be easier to attract two or three persons to share an apartment rather than five or more to share a large home. Lease stipulations may prevent apartment sharing; however, many successful arrangements have been made with landlords, and the agency's name is generally on the lease. If a sharer vacates the apartment, the agency is responsible for that person's portion of the rent until another tenant is found. Home sharers may lose entitlement benefits if their combined household income exceeds that necessary for eligibility. Sharing, as a cost-efficient option, can be encouraged through changes in regulatory and legislative language to remove eligibility benefit penalties.

Fannie Mae underwrites mortgages to develop the two home-sharing options. Some state housing agencies provide capital funds to community organizations to develop shared living for low- or mixed-income persons. Some state and local public agencies provide program operating funds. Mixed-income resident groups provide cross-subsidization for greater operating feasibility.

Because home-sharing programs are staff-intensive and serve a small segment of the elderly, funding sources often withdraw support in tight times, preferring to target efforts that show more outcome units per dollar spent. One strategy is to incorporate the home-sharing program within a general housing counseling service where total program units of service would be higher. Creative publicity campaigns and community forums have been successful in increasing consumers' and community leaders' awareness of these options and their benefits.

Because older people value privacy, many consider sharing only when living alone is no longer possible. Programs can fail when sponsors target younger well elderly and fail to include the staff/assistance required by the frail persons who become residents. Success depends upon agencies' understanding the market for these arrangements, as well as commitment to staff-intensive programming.

Rental Housing

The majority of rural rental senior housing is publicly funded as an affordable option for low-income elderly. Tenants are required to pay no more than 30% of their income for rent. Nonsubsidized senior rental housing attracts older persons seeking the convenience of a low-maintenance option that, in many cases, also includes supportive and health care services.

Rural rental housing developments are usually one- or two-story garden apartment complexes of 10 to 50 one-bedroom and studio units. These are typically located near population centers for easy access to services, activities, shopping, public transportation, etc. Projects' owners and managers often form liaisons with community service providers for access to congregate and home-delivered meals, supportive services, in-home care, transportation, and senior citizen activities.

The major federal funding sources for rural rental senior housing are the Farmers Home Administration's Section 515 capital loan program and the Department of Housing and Urban Development's Section 202 capital advance program. Other federal sources include the Federal National Mortgage Association and the Federal Home Loan Bank. Over the past decade, there has been increasing development of affordable rental housing by state and local housing development agencies to fill the gap left by the federal government's significant retrenchment in housing development. In the 1990 National Affordable Housing Act (NAHA), the federal government made a renewed commitment to the development of affordable housing. Under NAHA capital funds are allocated to state governments and local jurisdictions, with 15% of these funds reserved for Community Housing Development Organizations, many of which serve rural areas.

Local nonprofit development groups have access to federal Community Development Block Grant funds allocated to communities. Access to conventional financing has been enhanced for nonprofit groups by both the federal Community Reinvestment Act, which requires lending institutions to target low-income housing development, and by emerging community-based land trusts and loan funds that provide low-interest development loans to groups that have difficulty accessing traditional funding sources.

Benefits

Rental housing eliminates the maintenance and repair burdens of homeownership and provides an environment for social interaction when mobility and agility losses have reduced those opportunities. Older persons generally consider rental housing when frailty or financial instability compromises their ability to stay where they are. Because of increasing longevity and the trend of elderly homeowners to move into senior rental housing at older ages, these projects increasingly include on-site staff, congregate meals, social activities, housekeeping and transportation services, and facilitated access to personal care, thereby enhancing continued aging in place in the community. The aging of longtime residents in family rental housing has resulted in many of these projects evolving into naturally occurring retirement communities (NORCs). These are projects where 50% or more of residents are now aged 60 and older. The increasingly supportive environment of NORCs attracts other elderly who are seeking to relocate.

Barriers and Strategies

The predominant barrier to the development of rural rental housing is affordability. The sparsity of rural populations, the strong preference of rural elderly to remain in their family homes, and the pervasive poverty among rural elderly leave a small market for rental housing. The project size needed to respond to this small market is often not financially feasible to construct. Federal rental subsidies attached to the Section 515 Program to make these projects feasible are limited. Some states have developed state rental assistance programs to complement the federal subsidies, which has greatly enhanced utilization of the 515 Program. However, the remaining states still face the ongoing affordability issue. Other affordability strategies for rural senior rental housing include joint ventures of nonprofit and for-profit organizations to allow access to the federal Low-Income Housing Tax Credit program, unit clustering to reduce land costs, mixed-income resident groups to maximize cross-subsidization, use of manufactured housing options, and state-supported capital programs that subsidize specific cost areas such as infrastructure costs, predevelopment expenses, and communal space costs.

Integration of Multiunit Housing and Supportive Assistance

Over the past 15 years, the "aging-in-phenomenon" has resulted in the evolution of integrating housing and services for older people. A variety of successful integration strategies have been developed to accommodate the changing needs and preferences of aging persons and to address the added tasks assumed by housing managers to cope with the growing needs of these residents. As a basic response to aging in place, many owners have changed management practices for senior housing: They station the manager on-site within the housing project; they hire managers that have both traditional management skills and social work training; they hire from the growing number of firms that specialize in managing senior housing; and they provide their managers with professional training about the aging process, effective interaction with aging residents, and successful linkage with community services/agencies.

Increasingly, owners are hiring staff for their buildings as a complement to management, to perform such functions as linking needy residents with community services, coordinating service delivery to the building, acting as liaison with residents' families, counseling, information and referral, coordinating socialization activities, and providing case management. Such staff members are called service facilitators, service coordinators, resident advisers, tenant relations directors, etc. They may work full- or part-time, be professionals or paraprofessionals, live on- or off-site, and may include a resident-volunteer component for friendly visiting and informal monitoring of frail residents. In rural communities, several small developments sometimes use a circuit rider model, sharing the time and cost of a single facilitator; or an isolated small development that needs only part-time management can hire a full-time dual-trained person to both manage and perform the service facilitator functions.

Congregate housing is a housing and services integration strategy involving multiunit independent housing and including any of the following supportive services: housekeeping, homemaking, linen services, one to three congregate meals per day, transportation, shopping assistance, counseling, information and referral, personal care, and socialization activities. Services are provided by the development's own staff or are contracted from community agencies. Residents can buy services and meals on an as-used basis, or specific services can be included in the monthly rental charge, or services can be subsidized by public programs.

As the aging-in-phenomenon has grown, some owners have gradually converted their buildings into congregate housing by incrementally adding staff and meals/services/activities, with each development creating a unique model in response to its own resident profile. This ad hoc development has resulted in enormous creativity in customized program design.

Continuing care retirement communities (CCRCs) and life care communities (LCCs) represent the most comprehensive integration models, providing multiple levels of housing, supportive assistance, and health care. At a minimum, these complexes include independent living units (apartments or cottages); supportive services such as housekeeping, transportation, social activities, and congregate meals; and a skilled nursing facility. They may also include congregate apartments, assisted living units, in-home personal and nursing care, adult day care, and facilitated access to various therapies and medical care. The community's health care facilities can be located in separate buildings on the same campus as the housing or incorporated as a separate floor or wing of the independent living building. Communities may operate on traditional rental arrangements, as cooperatives, or under diverse long-term contractual arrangements guaranteeing housing and care.

As a nationwide industry, the planned-campus version of CCRCs and LCCs began about 25 years ago and has typically developed in rural and suburban areas because of the land space required for a campus arrangement and the market attractiveness of nonmetropolitan areas for retirement living. However, during this same period, in response to aging in place, versions of the continuing care concept have been developed incrementally in both rural and urban areas by sponsors who operate housing projects and health facilities in close proximity.

Benefits

The primary benefit of integrating housing and services is the availability of and facilitated access to the wide range of shelter and assistance residents need and want as they incur aging-related frailties. These strategies permit older people to exercise their first preference to age in place and delay or avoid institutionalization. Incorporating assistance and care within the independent living environment maximizes privacy and personal control over daily life during the frail years, two variables that are critical to life satisfaction among the elderly (Prosper, 1990b). Public policies that promote home care in place of institutional care for cost-containment purposes have changed the role and responsibilities of managers of housing with aging residents. Strategies that integrate housing and services address management's need for assistance in meeting this new role.

Barriers and Strategies

Although financially secure elderly can support the cost of on-site managers, service facilitators, and supportive services in monthly rents, developments for low- and moderate-income elderly must often rely on foundation grants, legislative seed monies, short-term public grants, community fund drives, and complex coordination with various public programs such as Medicaid, Supplemental Security Income, Administration on Aging programs, and state-supported in-home services programs. Also, still debated is the question of whether housing, aging, or health is responsible for such funding and whether nonmedical supportive and preventive assistance should be publicly supported. A limited number of states have developed state-subsidized congregate housing programs, and small congregate housing demonstration programs have been implemented by the Department of Housing and Urban Development and the Farmers Home Administration. Many state aging and housing agencies are funding service facilitator programs through demonstration grants from the R. W. Johnson Foundation and the Administration on Aging. In a collaborative pilot program by the New York State Office for the Aging, the state's Division of Housing and Community Renewal, and the Region II office of the U.S. Department of Housing and Urban Development, the cost of an on-site resident adviser is included in participating developments' operating budgets. HUD's redesigned Section 202 Program provides for the cost of a service coordinator and a portion of supportive services through the developments' Project Rental Assistance Contracts. Existing 202s can pay for service coordinators with the development's residual funds. HUD's Congregate Housing Services Program and HOPE for Elderly Independence Program integrate housing and services, dividing the costs between the federal housing network and the local community. All of these programs require or encourage collaboration between the housing and aging networks to capitalize on both systems' expertise and resources.

Rural rental projects are relatively small and rural homeowners are scattered, making staffing and service delivery costly. Case management and service coordination models that are collaboratively planned and jointly funded by several community aging, health, housing, and service agencies have been developed in rural areas as financially efficient strategies for meeting the needs of both homeowners and renters. The addition of congregate housing units can be a logical extension of rural nursing homes and hospitals, creating a continuum-of-care option for residents and an economic development opportunity for the health care facilities.

Although new residents are attracted to the supportive environment of an integrated housing/services development, owners will often encounter resistance to the introduction of services and staff by longtime residents who fear that their independent housing will take on the character of a nursing home. Incremental development, as well as resident education and involvement in decision making and program planning, can mediate this resistance.

Rural elderly traits of independence and self-sufficiency create resistance to relocating from family homes into rental housing developed in adjacent villages and cities. At the same time, affluent urban retirees may find a rural retirement development initially attractive but may become disenchanted by the lack of public transportation, slower-paced environment, and reduced access to the diversity of shops and cultural activities found in large cities. Developers for both groups find greater marketing success by attending to elderly consumer preferences, adequately defining and targeting a population that both needs and wants the intended housing and services, and matching the previous lifestyles and surroundings of the intended resident population.

Policy and Research Issues

The demographics of aging have spurred an enormous amount of research on the older population. Housing-specific research has focused primarily on the impact of the living environment on older persons' physical and psychological well-being during the later years, the issue of provision of long-term care in housing versus institutional environments, and the capacity of various housing options to maximize older persons' privacy, personal control, and ability to continue living in the community. As the housing environment assumes greater importance as the locus for providing social, supportive, and health care assistance in the later years, several policy and research areas warrant greater attention.

First, the trends in longevity and in the integration of housing and services have been accompanied by a concomitant emergence of ethical and liability issues for housing owners, service providers, and both well and frail elderly tenants. Such issues include individual rights, tenants' rights, self-determination regarding health care and safety issues, relocation procedures, quality of care, abuse/victimization, locus of legal responsibility for injury, imposition of a regulatory framework, and so on. Meshing the traditional housing environment with a health care environment interweaves real property and landlord/tenant law with health care law. Increasing attention is warranted in defining rights, responsibilities, and avenues for redress of all interested parties regarding the provision of assistance and health care in housing environments.

Second, policy, program, and housing developers seek to match needs and preferences with options and choice in order to achieve appropriate levels/costs of assistance, maximum quality of life for older persons, and market share. To achieve these goals, much greater emphasis must be placed on accurately defining the diverse housing/services needs and preferences of the many subgroups that make up the older population:

age segments, gender, family circumstances, socioeconomic status, cultural heritage and lifestyle, geographic location, income status, functional capacity, etc.

Third, demographic, preference, and policy trends continue to promote the integration of housing and long-term care. A variety of practice-based models are needed that demonstrate creative financing mechanisms for providing housing and services as an alternative to facility-based care. These include long-term care insurance or Medicaid coverage of preventive and supportive assistance services; mixing income populations in public housing; tax credits and vouchers for caregiving families; capital funding for design and architectural needs to create dementia wings in housing projects; collaborative sharing of resources among health, aging, housing, and family networks; public-private partnerships; and joint ventures by nonprofit and for-profit organizations.

Fourth, many rural areas have experienced extended periods of economic decline that have affected all aspects and all age groups in the community. Although strategies that address the needs of one sector often resolve the needs of another, providers typically define and address discrete problem areas in isolation. Successful planning models that demonstrate a collaborative communitywide approach to problem solving and resource use must be identified and described for replication. Such models clarify the interwoven links between a community's private and public sectors, between its formal and informal networks, and among its employment, housing, health care, economic development, education, overall families' needs, and so on.

Summary and Conclusions

Rural older householders are predominantly homeowners. Their first preference is to age where they are and never move. However, the physical and mental frailties and financial instability associated with advancing age compromise their ability to age in place viably. The circumstances that render the housing environment inappropriate vary dramatically among the elderly because housing suitability is related to the physical condition and location of the house as well as the health, financial status, family circumstances, age, culture, lifestyle, and preferences unique to each person. In addition, needs and preferences change during the aging process, and the housing environment must flexibly adapt to meet these changes.

Policy makers, aging advocates, service providers, and housing sponsors have responded to the aging-in-phenomenon place by (a) developing a variety of programs that make an older person's existing housing safe, secure, affordable, physically adaptable, and accommodating to changing needs; (b) creating a variety of housing models that permit older consumers greater choice in alternatives; and (c) increasing the diverse services that provide in-home and community-based supportive assistance and health care. Choice is the key to creating viable living environments that are responsive to the diversity found among the elderly population.

In rural areas, community planning for older persons' housing needs cannot occur in isolation. Rather, such planning is directly tied to planning for the needs of the total community. A collaborative community-wide partnership that includes public and private sectors, various community agencies, and the informal network can maximize the benefits for all groups, as well as rebuild the intergenerational support system and sense of community that traditionally typify rural areas.

The demographics of aging have brought recognition to the changing role that housing plays in the long-term care needs of older people and have focused research attention and practice-based efforts on the elderly and their families. Research efforts must expand to include the growing ethical implications of providing supportive assistance and health care in the home environment, the demonstration of community partnership efforts in meeting housing and care needs, and greater emphasis on defining the changing needs and preferences of subsegments of an increasingly aging population. Advocates and policy makers can use these findings and models to garner continuing support for creating the most appropriate and viable living environments for all elderly persons.

8

Respite and Adult Day Care for Rural Elders

VICKI L. SCHMALL
LINDA COOK WEBB

Providing care to a frail or impaired family member can be all-consuming and can take its toll on the caregiver. One caregiver, age 70, stated:

> I have taken care of my husband for three years. Each day is a "36-hour day." I am exhausted. It's hard to even get out and get food and his medicine. I always enjoyed my home, but now I feel trapped. . . . My home has become a prison.

Caregivers often report chronic fatigue, role conflict, isolation, family turmoil, financial stress, and declining physical and mental health (Sharlach & Frenzel, 1986). Some older persons are placed in care facilities not because of deterioration in their health, but because of deterioration in the health—and sometimes the death—of their caregivers (Butler & Newacheck, 1981). The need for relief from the continuous demands and stress of caregiving has been well documented (see, e.g., Anthony-Bergstone, Zarit, & Gatz, 1988; Zarit & Teri, 1991). Without breaks, the stresses inherent in continuous caregiving can lead to neglect or abuse of the care recipient.

156

Respite and adult day care programs can provide caregivers with much-needed breaks in caregiving, giving them time to pursue personal interests and activities and to take care of other business, thus enabling them to continue providing care. In rural areas, however, such programs often are not available. When they do exist, program use is often limited by geographic isolation and the tendency of rural individuals to use the informal support system of family and friends.

Scope, Nature, and Need for Services

Respite means "relief" or "time off." The purpose of respite care is to provide planned temporary or periodic relief to informal caregivers— primarily family members, but also friends and neighbors providing continuous care or supervision to a frail, dependent person—to prevent their emotional and physical exhaustion. Another common goal is the encouragement of family support of the frail elderly, and thus prevention or delay of institutional care (Rosenheimer & Francis, 1992). Respite care may be provided in or out of the home. It may be provided on a planned or emergency basis, for a few hours a day, as day care or overnight care, or for weekends or periods of a week or longer.

The primary intended beneficiary of respite services is the caregiver rather than the care receiver. However, in many cases, the respite provider may represent the only opportunity the care receiver has for out-side-the-family socialization. The care receiver also benefits from a caregiver's being "refreshed" following a break in caregiving ("Evidence Mounts," 1990). Also, respite care that involves temporary admission to a care facility can provide a positive opportunity for reviewing and changing the medication regimen of a care receiver (Meltzer, 1982).

Adult day care often provides respite to caregivers; however, it differs in focus from what we refer to here as *respite care*. Adult day care brings frail and impaired persons into a congregate setting with a group of their peers. It promotes participants' optimum level of functioning through individualized plans of care and provides socialization, stimulation with peers, and activities targeted to their level. Adult day care also differs from respite in that it is provided outside the home and never for a full 24-hour period (National Institute on Adult Day Care, 1990; Webb, 1989).

Standard and Alternative Approaches to Programming

Respite and adult day care develop uniquely in every rural community, depending on the specific needs and resources available. Specific types of programs cover a wide range of service patterns, locations, and sponsoring agencies. The following categories are a sample of traditional and alternative programs implemented by rural communities.

Respite Programs

Respite can take many forms, ranging from help in the home for a few hours a week to placing the frail older person in a nursing home for a limited time. The various types of respite programs and their advantages and disadvantages are reviewed by Rathbone-McCuan and Coward (1985). Some types of respite programs are described below.

Companion sitter programs. These programs provide respite in the home. Frequently, sitters are provided only for one or two half-days per week, with the goal of giving short, regular breaks to the caregiver. While in the home, the sitter visits with, reads to, or writes letters for the frail person. The sitter may serve a simple meal and remind a disoriented care receiver when to go to the bathroom. Sitters are trained in how to respond to basic emergencies, but they do not give medications or provide personal care.

Companion sitter programs are ideally suited to rural areas because of the relatively small number of potential clients and their geographic spread. It is often easier and less expensive to send a companion into the home than to transport the disabled person over long distances. Companion sitters may be regular paid staff, staff subsidized through senior employment programs, or volunteers.

Volunteer caregiver respite programs. These programs are often organized through interfaith programs, health departments, or visiting nurses' associations. Volunteers generally "adopt" specific families and provide a range of respite services. In addition to sitter services, they are trained to provide telephone reassurance, escorted transportation, shopping assistance, friendly visiting, chore assistance, and help in locating resources. Volunteers are supported by in-service training and consultation with nurses and/or social workers.

Overnight respite. Overnight respite can be provided by a sitter in the home, but it is most frequently offered in nursing homes or hospitals that have available beds. The impaired person is brought to the facility for a predetermined length of time—usually for less than two weeks, but possibly longer. This option is often used by caregivers around harvest time or to allow visits to ill family members in another town. Services provided are much like those offered to regular nursing home residents.

The short-term nature of a respite program can present unique challenges to care facilities (Miller, Gulle, & McCue, 1986). The required paperwork can be overwhelming, there often is not enough time for staff to become familiar with the needs of a short-term resident, and staff patterns and assignments often need to be adjusted, which may be disruptive for both staff and residents, particularly those in small facilities. For certain frail older people, particularly those afflicted with Alzheimer's disease, it can be difficult to adapt to a strange environment in a short time. Evidence suggests that it is best for a care facility to assign respite patients to a designated unit, rather than to whatever beds are vacant. However, it is more costly to maintain a designated respite unit, so this may not be feasible for most care facilities in rural communities.

Adult Day Care

Adult day care is a generic term that applies to a variety of programs with services that may range from social activities to health-related services to rehabilitation. Some centers may emphasize particular directions of service by calling themselves "day activities," "adult day health care," or "day treatment" centers. In the past, the terms *social model* and *medical model* were used to try to distinguish types of centers. In practice, it is difficult to identify any given center as falling into either category. All centers have social components, and all provide some degree of health services. For this reason, the National Institute on Adult Day Care (1984, 1990) uses voluntary standards that discuss the range of services that can be provided in adult day care, not *models*. However, the *model* terminology does remain in a few states that make distinctions in service packages for Medicaid reimbursement purposes or licensing regulations.

Most adult day care programs serve mixed populations in terms of age and impairment, but some serve special populations. An ongoing debate has to do with providing services to special populations such as persons with Alzheimer's disease, head injury, sensory deficits, mental retardation, AIDS, or mental illness. On one side is the argument that specialized centers can more fully train their staffs to meet the needs of these persons. In contrast is the position that a generalist center empowers participants by allowing each to find someone he or she can help. In a small community, the generalist center may be the only practical program. Many of these centers have developed parallel programming to allow for attention to be given to individuals with special needs during a part of each day. Under the right circumstances, both specialized and generalist services can be done well.

The National Institute on Adult Day Care (1990) has written voluntary standards that outline eight essential services of adult day care: personal care, nursing services, social services, therapeutic activities, nutrition and therapeutic diets, transportation, emergency care for participants, and family education. Additional services often include physical, occupational, and speech therapy; baths; cosmetologist or barber visits; dentistry; podiatry; pharmacy; psychological services; and eye care, audiology, or other medical services.

Adult day care centers may be freestanding, but most are located within other agencies. If a building is shared with another service, day care should have its own designated space and staff. The range of adult day care programs is rather wide; several types are discussed below (Webb & Heide, 1991).

Church-based adult day care. Churches often cosponsor or operate adult day centers with other agencies, such as Area Agencies on Aging, health departments, or local colleges. These centers tend to focus on providing supervision and promoting socialization in a friendly environment. The rural church can be an ideal location. It is generally known to many potential participants, has space available for weekday use, and may have a kitchen for preparing meals. The congregation may view adult day care as a special ministry and thus may be a ready source for volunteers and donations. A church-based center usually needs extra storage space and physical flexibility to allow it to convert back to a fellowship hall or Sunday school rooms once a week.

Senior center-based adult day care. Some rural senior centers report that they "backed into" adult day care because they found themselves providing more and more supportive services to center members. The sensitivity of management is critical, because healthier center members sometimes feel threatened by the introduction of adult day care. Not only does adult day care usually reduce the space available for traditional programming, but members may be forced to confront their own fears of frailty. On the other hand, members may be encouraged when they see the benefits of day care for their friends who need special help and may be glad that assistance will be available to them, if needed.

Nursing home-based adult day care. Because health care providers are limited in rural areas, developing adult day care in a nursing home can be cost-effective in regard to both staffing and finances. Persons who have severe physical disabilities can be offered therapy, baths, podiatry, dentistry, and many special services already in place in the nursing home. The nursing home can also share dietary, social services, laundry, and some activities.

Nursing home-based adult day care centers face some special challenges. Potential participants may be reluctant to visit the adult day center because they fear being "dumped" in a nursing home. A separate entrance can help reduce this perception. Conducting intake evaluations at participants' homes is also helpful. This gives the program director a chance to develop rapport and to explain the separate nature of the center. A short visit at the center can complete the admission. During this visit, the applicant can talk with current participants and learn that participants do go home at night.

Hospital-based adult day care. Adult day care centers based in hospitals tend to be the most focused toward physical rehabilitation and nursing services. There are likely to be natural referral patterns when persons are discharged from the hospital and still need therapy or professional supervision. In hospitals that have reduced census and are seeking a new focus in services, adult day care can be an excellent use of space. When they combine adult day care with swing beds and/or overnight respite, hospitals can provide a continuum of long-term care.

In locations where they still exist, rural hospitals are such hubs of health care that community acceptance of a hospital-based center should be high. With the closing of rural hospitals continuing, however, income is a great concern. Adult day care does not generate substantial revenues; therefore, fewer rural hospitals may be interested in providing this service. Another option could be for a hospital to cosponsor adult day care with another agency, thus sharing the risk and maximizing benefits.

Portable adult day care. Efforts to develop adult day care centers in rural areas often have not been successful because of a limited client base and the cost of transporting clients long distances. Portable adult day care is a creative option for rural areas in which there is no significant concentration of potential participants. Satellite centers, each open one or more days per week, are established throughout the area to be served. Locations can include churches, American Legion halls, schools, or any facility with sufficient space. Staff, and possibly even small equipment and supplies, then rotate days at each location. In the beginning, the entire staff may serve multiple locations. As the program grows, it might be just the professional staff who rotate. These satellite sites reduce or eliminate the need to transport care recipients over long distances (Gunter, 1985).

Adult day care homes. Adult day care homes—private family homes providing care for one to four persons—are another nontraditional response to rural needs (Goldston, 1985). They have the potential for serving persons within their neighborhoods and communities. Several states—including Hawaii, Idaho, Maine, New Mexico, North Carolina, and North Dakota—have such confidence in this option that they have written regulations for the provision and Medicaid reimbursement of adult day care in homes. The National Institute on Adult Day Care (1990) standards discuss special requirements for adult day care homes.

Running an adult day care home is not like "having four grandmas who come to visit." It is a hard job. Providers usually receive low pay considering the disruption they may experience in family life. Providers most interested in operating adult day care homes may not have the skills for caring for confused or disabled persons, and they can become isolated and overburdened by a very demanding situation. States in which adult day care homes have worked well offer a great deal of support to providers to combat these problems. Having the county welfare/social services office, health department, or a central adult day care center do admissions, reassessments, and discharges ensures that participants are matched with appropriate environments. In-service education and peer support through state associations also reduce isolation and increase the skill levels among providers.

Because potential providers often have unrealistic perceptions about what it means to operate an adult day care home, an orientation program for potential providers is critical. An orientation should provide a realistic view of a day in the life of an adult day care home provider, characteristics of participants, and the range of problems and issues providers sometimes face.

Developing and Providing Services:
Problems and Solutions

One issue that rural program planners confront is that sometimes the solution becomes bigger than the problem. Usually, a new program comes about because someone has heard about a good program done elsewhere. People get excited about the concept and want it for their own area. Others agree and a new program is born. However, a program that works well across the state may not necessarily address local needs.

Many rural programs have failed because planners did not first ensure that they had the right structure for meeting their community needs. Listening to local people describe their needs can prove quite enlightening. They often surprise program planners with the simplicity of their desires. Families know that they want a break from responsibility, time to themselves, peace of mind, and the knowledge that Mom is happy and receiving quality care. Those are the things they need. Respite programs and adult day care centers are merely structures for meeting those needs.

Although respite and adult day care have many benefits, developing and sustaining such programs is not always easy. Challenges encountered in rural areas include the following (Gunter, 1985):

- *Low population density:* The population base is small and spread across a large geographic area. For example, a service area may cover 10 counties and 800 square miles with a population of only 15,000 people.
- *Transportation:* Travel distances and costs of transportation are generally higher for both staff and clients.
- *Low informal support:* There is an absence of linkages with the informal support network.
- *Low formal support:* There is a lack of linkages with the formal health and social service systems.

Because of geographic distances and sparse populations, traditional adult day care centers may not be the best response in some rural areas. In some communities, it may be best to start with a companion sitter respite program. In other areas, where resources are stretched to the breaking point, it may be better to start with a telephone reassurance program. In any event, direction should be taken from the people to be served.

Barriers to Families Using Programs

Even when respite and adult day care programs exist, families often do not take advantage of them. Some of the barriers to access and use are discussed below.

Lack of awareness. Families often are not aware of the availability of respite or adult day care or program eligibility, or they may not be familiar with the provider agency (MaloneBeach, Zarit, & Spore, 1992). Many caregiving families have had little or no contact with service agencies (Montgomery & Borgatta, 1989). In some rural areas, the distances and isolation of rural living further contribute to a lack of awareness of services that do exist.

Knowledge, whether individual or prescriptive, seems to be a predictor of the use of adult day care. Beisecker and Wright (1991) found that lack of knowledge was a significant barrier to the use of adult day care by both user and nonuser caregivers. Almost 20% of the caregivers who used adult day care cited knowing about it as being partially responsible for their having used it, and 25% indicated that they had been told to use the service. Finding a sympathetic person within the service system as well as having information about service availability and eligibility may affect the use of community-based services (MaloneBeach et al., 1992).

Apprehension. With in-home respite, some caregivers are apprehensive about leaving family members with "strangers" or nonprofessional care providers, or are mistrustful of outsiders (Miller & Goldman, 1989). They may also be afraid that their impaired family members will interpret their leaving as evidence of a lack of caring (Dunn, 1988).

Attitudes. Caregivers have differing attitudes toward the use of respite and adult day care. Some caregivers are fiercely independent, taking the stance that "I can [or should be able to] care for my family member myself," or "No one can care for him/her as I can." Others feel it is selfish to meet their own needs, feel guilt at leaving their family members in the care of someone else, or believe that using formal services is a sign of failure (Netting & Kennedy, 1985; "Reaching the Caregiver," 1992; Rosenheimer & Francis, 1992). As a result, they are reluctant to accept help. It is often useful to reinforce with caregivers that a need for a break in caregiving is not a reflection of inadequacy on their part.

Beisecker and Wright (1991) found that having negative feelings toward using any respite was the second most common reason caregivers gave for not using adult day care. Caregivers in their sample either felt that adult day care had no benefit or did not perceive their family members as being "at the right stage" for adult day care.

A challenge sometimes encountered in rural areas has to do with common client personalities. There may be a tendency for rural persons to reject anything perceived as new, untried, unfamiliar, or foreign, particularly if it has any overtones of charity. One successful method for removing the stigma attached to adult day care centers is to develop a scrapbook of pictures from "a day at the center." When potential client families recognize some of the faces in the pictures, they may feel more comfortable with the concept of adult day care. This also subtly gives them the chance to ask current participants and their families about the center. (It should be noted that one must gain the permission of any clients photographed before using their pictures in this way.)

Timing. Respite services are most beneficial when used early in the caregiving process, as a preventive measure to reduce caregiver burnout. Many caregivers, however, view respite as a last resort. They seek services much too late—when they are in crisis, desperate, or the impaired family member is severely debilitated and requires heavy care beyond what respite or adult day care can provide (Montgomery & Borgatta, 1989). In part, this may be because many publicly funded programs limit access to those families providing care to persons "at risk of institutionalization." According to Dunn (1988), the message frequently given to caregivers is: "Respite is a service when you are having trouble coping or the condition of your loved one is progressing to the point where placement [in a care facility] may be necessary" (p. 2). Therefore, some caregivers may look at respite as a program meant to *treat* physical and emotional exhaustion, rather than to *prevent* it.

Finances. Some caregivers are unwilling to use or delay the use of respite or adult day care because of the costs of services or anticipated future health care costs. Questions that caregivers frequently ask themselves include the following: If I spend money on respite for myself, will I have the money needed later for hospital or nursing home care for my spouse? How can I afford day care for my mother and still pay my children's college bills? Other caregivers are not willing to pay for programs they view as "baby-sitting services." Another barrier for some who wish to use respite and day care services is the fact that Medicare and most private insurance companies do not provide reimbursement (Deimling, 1989; Van Werkhooven, 1991-1992).

Characteristics and reactions of the care recipient. Some studies suggest that care recipients, especially those with cognitive impairment and low morale, resist respite care more than do their caregivers (Geiser, Hoche, & King, 1988; Gonyea, 1988). Negative reactions of a care receiver may include resentment about someone coming into the home, about the caregiver leaving, or about having a "baby-sitter." This resistance may be the reason a caregiver does not use respite or day care. In other cases, the care recipient may be too impaired for the service or may be unwilling or unable to endure lengthy travel time to get to the service (Deimling, 1989; Gunter, 1985).

Problems in getting the care recipient ready and transporting him or her to a center constitute another factor limiting the use of adult day care by some caregivers (Ehrlich & White, 1991). Also, caregivers sometimes feel that care is less disruptive when it is provided in the home. As one caregiver said, "The time and energy required to get my husband ready for the day care program just was not worth it." Berry, Zarit, and Rabatin (1991) found that caregivers who used adult day care services actually spent more time performing caregiving activities on respite days than on nonrespite days. The explanation was that preparing the care recipient to leave the home was more time-consuming and exhausting than the usual care.

System inflexibility and bureaucracy. Program inflexibility or perceived inflexibility may also contribute to lower usage of respite and adult day care programs. System barriers reported by caregivers include the following (MaloneBeach et al., 1992):

- lack of service availability when it is most wanted or needed, for example, on evenings or weekends
- accommodation only of older persons with a "narrow band of need"; persons with behavioral and emotional problems or with more severe functional impairment are often ineligible
- lack of responsiveness in the service system, especially when level of service is changed only on a fixed schedule rather than in response to changes in the older person's functioning
- lack of a system whereby caregivers can preselect or specify particular workers (Caregivers tend to prefer the dependability of one respite worker to whom they can relate over time, rather than different workers each time they request help; Meltzer, 1982.)
- having to make a series of calls to arrange for respite care, services not being provided as had been arranged, and other inefficiencies in the system

For some caregivers, perceived control may be an important factor in whether or not they use services. Caregivers generally want some control in regard to when and by whom in-home services are provided (MaloneBeach et al., 1992). Making sure that services are "caregiver friendly" may be a critical factor in their acceptance and use.

Service delivery. Respite and adult day care face special problems in rural areas. Some counties have had no health professionals for years. One rural Maryland adult day center, for example, has to pay extra mileage to professional staff who live in neighboring counties. This can place undue budgetary pressure on a program that may, at best, break even. The most recent National Institute on Adult Day Care (1990) standards discuss ways adult day care should be modified in rural areas. Recommendations include the following:

- sharing professional staff with other agencies
- increasing the role of paraprofessionals
- substituting experience for education in staff background
- changing state practices acts
- sharing facilities or developing day care homes

Respite and adult day care should be embedded in a larger system of care, for example, linked to a case management system (Brody, Saperstein, & Lawton, 1989; Meltzer, 1982). Brody et al. (1989) found that half of the caregivers in their study needed and received referrals to other agencies for services such as medical care, legal services, transportation, and self-help groups; 60% received counseling, mostly short-term; and two-thirds required and received education. According to Berry et al. (1991), respite should be a "service package" that includes assessment of need, education, respite, and follow-up.

Funding. Financial stability is a major issue for respite and adult day care programs. No matter how needed or how well planned, most new programs struggle financially for the first few years (Henry, 1992). Most programs that go under do so within five years of opening. Programs that survive financial losses have boards of directors, administrators, staff, and communities who have faith in the program's mission. That faith is then carried out in long-range planning. The long-range plan may cover only one year at a time, but it has specific action steps to bring the program measurably closer to its goals. As steps are implemented, they are evaluated, and the plan is adapted as necessary. The real secret, as one director put it, is to "believe, believe, believe."

Funding is a chronic problem in adult day care. Because of the nature of participants' physical and mental conditions, close supervision and some professional involvement is needed. Facilities must be adapted so that they are accessible to disabled individuals. Special transportation should be offered. All of this costs money. In contrast, respite and adult day care programs must be affordable, to encourage use at the time when they can have the most benefit. In many states, Medicaid reimburses adult day care, but only for the most impoverished persons. Medicare and most private insurers do not pay at all. This leaves many potential participants unable to afford the programs.

Sliding fee scales and scholarship funds can help low- and middle-income families with extensive medical expenses to afford services (Deimling, 1989). Traditional sources of funding to support reduced costs to families include the following:

- Title IIIB and IIID of the Older Americans Act (contact the Area Agency on Aging)
- Title XX of the Social Security Act (Medicaid)
- county funds for senior citizens or the handicapped
- employment programs that subsidize salaries for staff in training
- foundation grants
- private insurance, particularly if there is coverage for long-term care
- individual donations
- fund-raising events
- donations of facilities, staff, equipment, or supplies from other agencies

Successful adult day centers use all of these funds, combined with full or partial payment from families. Within families, there may also be opportunities for flexibility. If the caregiver cannot afford the service, there may be another family member who can. Family members who live at a distance are sometimes able and willing to help financially even though they are unable to provide direct care. Some centers even bill a patchwork of four or more sources for a single participant. For example, three family members may each pay one day per week, a Title IIIB contract for scholarships picks up one day, and a privately funded "scholarship" pays one day.

For a center to stay open, costs must be covered. The Dementia and Respite Services Program has shown that programs achieving financial self-sufficiency do the following (Henry, 1992):

- Market aggressively and continuously.
- Charge what services cost.
- Increase the volume—that is, use—of services. This lowers the unit cost. In a rural area, however, the volume simply may not be available.
- Use a prepayment system for services in which caregivers pay in advance for days scheduled for the month as opposed to paying for actual days used. Prepayment can increase revenue and consistency of program use by reducing late cancellations.
- Employ a variety of strategies.

Transportation. Transportation is a major issue, particularly for adult day care centers. Many participants need handicapped-accessible or escorted transportation. Few families are able to provide such transportation, and public senior transportation systems may not be available or may already be operating at capacity. It is also expensive to provide special transportation. Many centers patch together systems that include families, senior citizen van services, and vehicles borrowed from other agencies; some purchase their own vans.

Transportation is a special problem in rural areas because of the relatively greater distances to be traveled. Most standards and regulations state that adult day care participants should be in transit no more than one hour, yet some older people may live two hours away from available services. Creative directors have solved this problem in a couple of ways. Some use cars instead of vans. For the cost of one van, a center can get two station wagons. The drivers are trained to transfer participants into the vehicles and to fold wheelchairs down to fit in the back. By picking up fewer persons per run and doubling the number of vehicles, a center can cut transport time. Some centers break up lengthy trips with "rest stops" at restaurants. Others send an activities aide who conducts sing-alongs, word games, and discussion groups in the vehicle. The trip is still just as long, but distraction helps the time pass pleasantly. This method also has the added advantage of providing a second staff person in the event of an emergency.

Providers of in-home respite in rural areas often find that a large share of their time is spent traveling from one place to the next. Organizing services so as to reduce travel time of providers and yet still meet the scheduling needs of families who desire or need respite can be a major challenge. In some rural areas, families also have to travel long distances to use institution-based respite care programs.

Program flexibility. Flexibility is critical to the viability of programs in rural areas, especially in responding to changes in community needs and resources (Gunter, 1985). For example, during a recession, enrollments often drop. A recession can also affect fund-raising and the ability of families to pay for services. Programs that develop a variety of funding sources increase their ability to respond to these situations.

Flexibility is also needed in daily operations. Both respite and adult day care serve frail people whose conditions can change dramatically and quickly. As Netting and Kennedy (1985) state, "Changes that occur within these [caregiving] households are often erratic and rapid. Levels of family burden or client functioning can change daily" (p. 575). The more flexible a program, the more responsive it can be to changes in a caregiver's need and a care recipient's level of functioning. Staff should be flexible enough to deal with these changes, and program administrators should provide staff with needed support to cope with the stress that sometimes occurs.

Programs need to be customer driven in services offered, such as expanded hours, transportation, and in-home services. An employed caregiver who needs day care from 7:30 a.m. until 5:30 p.m. will find it difficult to use a program if its hours of operation are only from 9:00 to 3:00. Guiding practice principles in developing consumer-focused services should be caregiver autonomy, minimal professional intervention, and system flexibility in responding to the changing needs of the caregiver ("First Program," 1992).

Ease of program use. Rules, regulations, and/or practices can make it easy or difficult for clients to use a program. Caregivers who feel they are getting the runaround or who believe a program will place greater demands on them in terms of time, energy, or money are less receptive to what a program has to offer (Montgomery & Borgatta, 1989). The last thing a caregiver wants is another hassle, whether that be in getting information, making application, or using a program. If a caregiver must give detailed personal and financial information to meet eligibility requirements, he or she may consider this an intrusion of privacy and therefore may not apply. For in-home respite, caregivers want reliable and consistent providers. Each time a new person comes in to provide respite, the caregiver must spend time and energy to educate the respite worker about the care situation.

Staffing. Staff members are the backbone of good respite and adult day care programs. They are the people who are seen by clients and who provide the service. A person's perception of the staff will determine to a large degree his or her perception of the program or service. Unfortunately, qualified staff members can be difficult to find in rural areas, and when found, they seldom can be highly rewarded financially. This makes it even more important to find nonmonetary rewards for staff.

Staff loyalty can be cultivated in many ways. Directors can make a point of complimenting staff members on a job well done, especially in front of other staff, clients, or people from the community. They can also motivate staff by encouraging them to increase their skill levels through in-service education, reading, or workshops. Ironically, increased roles and responsibilities can also motivate staff. Paraprofessional staff usually welcome a blurring of the distinctions between their roles and those of professional staff. For example, a sitter can be trained to watch for newly developing care needs and to assist the family in seeking resources.

Training of providers is essential for a quality program. Providers need to understand the medical and emotional issues of care recipients; to have skills in relating to elders with special needs, such as persons with Alzheimer's disease; and to be sensitive to the needs and stresses of family caregivers (Meltzer, 1982). Ongoing training and supervision also contribute to staff retention. If a program relies heavily on volunteers, it is important that administrators recognize the amount of professional time necessary to operate a quality volunteer program. All too often, the time needed to train and support volunteers is underestimated.

Marketing. Marketing is a major challenge. Respite and adult day care are still relatively new in the United States, being just over 20 years old. In many rural areas, the concept of these services is still unknown. Caregivers often lack information about respite or adult day care and when and how these programs can help them. Ideally, respite care should be preventive, rather than crisis oriented. We need to help caregivers recognize that caregiving is a job and that the need for respite begins with the onset of caregiving. Just as employees benefit from regular breaks and vacations, caregivers, too, benefit from being able to take breaks from their job.

One particularly important challenge is how to reach caregivers who could benefit from respite and adult day care and enlist their participation. Montgomery and Borgatta (1989) have found that the mass media—television, radio, and newspapers—are a primary way to reach caregivers. However, dissemination of messages through the mass media can be problematic, because it relies on individuals to identify themselves as caregivers in need of services.

The message presented to caregivers may be particularly important. Traditionally, marketing has stressed the benefits of respite and adult day care for the caregiver. However, many caregivers are reluctant to use services for themselves. One study found that caregivers who perceived adult day care as primarily benefiting the caregiver were less likely to use the service than were caregivers who viewed adult day care as beneficial primarily for the person receiving care (Beisecker & Wright, 1991). Care-receiver benefits need to be documented and shared with caregivers and providers. It is likely that the resistance of some caregivers to respite and adult day care would decrease if they received more messages emphasizing how programs benefit care recipients.

The best way to market respite or adult day care is still unclear. Based on their study of caregivers, Lawton, Brody, and Saperstein (1989b) conclude, "If services are to be made more effective, they must speak to the needs of families who are potential targets of such services" (p. 34). These authors note that marketing must emphasize not only how programs relieve burden, but also how they reinforce caregiver satisfaction. They suggest the following ways to increase the appeal of respite to caregivers:

- Portray respite as a normal type of help that is beneficial to anyone, even the most successful of caregivers.
- Emphasize how respite helps to maintain the positive aspects of caregiving.
- Reassure caregivers that they deserve time off and are not deserting their family members by taking breaks from caregiving.

Because caregivers' needs, problems, and motivations vary, multiple marketing strategies may be important. According to findings from the Caregiver Market Segmentation Project of the Dementia Care and Respite Services Project, it is probably a mistake to design just one promotional message for reaching caregivers ("Reaching the Caregiver," 1992). Targeted messages will likely be more effective in actually getting people to use respite and adult day care. The Caregiver Market Segmentation Project identified five market segments, each of which is attracted to services for different reasons: "information seekers," "respite seekers: the givers," "respite seekers: the responsibles," "care seekers: the delegators," and "care seekers: the balancers."

Marketing also needs to speak the language of the group to which a program is being marketed. Not all people know the meaning of the term *respite,* and not all caregivers identify themselves as *caregivers.* Also, the times at which people begin to identify themselves as caregivers vary. For example, Montgomery and Borgatta (1989) found that "children end their caregiving careers at about the time spouses begin identifying themselves as caregivers" (p. 463).

Program names can sometimes be more important than people realize. The term *day care* can be a barrier because some people equate it with taking care of children (Bane, 1992). As one caregiver said, "The greatest mistake I made was talking with my mother using the term *day care*. Her response was, 'I am not a child.' " Caregivers and care receivers may be more receptive to programs with such names as "St. Aiden's Place" or "The Grace Center" than to any services including or emphasizing *day care* in the program name or marketing efforts. Adult day care center directors indicate that this also gives caregivers more flexibility in talking with their older family members about the programs; they can use more acceptable expressions, perhaps discussing going to "the club" or the "senior center."

Sometimes it is difficult to get caregivers to come in just to visit a program. One adult day center in Oregon found that it was important to take information out to families rather than expecting families to come in. A videotape was developed showing a variety of center activities as well as caregivers, professionals, and participants talking about how the center had enhanced the lives of participants. The videotape is mailed to families who call about the center and has been placed in the offices of physicians, service agencies, and the local hospital. Enrollment in the day care program has increased significantly since the videotape was produced. Such visual presentations should be positive. As one center director said, "You must show your best; otherwise, it's easy for people to say, 'My mother's not that bad.' " Some centers also offer potential client families one or two free days to bring their family members to the center to "try out" the program.

It is not enough to get the message out once and then just do an excellent job of service. People typically do not hear messages about respite or adult day care until they themselves need such services. Therefore, programs continually have to tell the community what they can do.

The referral system. People often make judgments about a program based not only on the quality of the information they receive, but on their opinions about the sources of that information. A trusted referral source—for example, a physician, clergy member, hospital, or agency—can be important in validating the need for and use of respite and adult day care services ("Reaching the Caregiver," 1992). Information that comes from a trusted family member, a respected newspaper columnist or radio announcer, or a support group may be considered of higher quality than the same information found in a newspaper advertisement (Montgomery, 1992).

Reaching caregivers directly is important, but outreach efforts should include targeting agencies and professionals who have contact with caregivers and providing them with information about respite and adult day care and how to access programs. Miller et al. (1986) recommends talking with potential referral sources and leaving brief written information about a program so that the professional can refer to it later and share it with caregivers. Outreach efforts also should be directed to potential "gatekeepers" in the community, such as pharmacists, who may fill prescriptions for both care receivers and caregivers and are in a position to observe changes in caregivers and to talk with them about the need for assistance.

Marketing to referral sources should include clear messages about funding and the flexibility of funding. Sometimes major referral sources may be convinced that their clients cannot afford to pay anything toward the cost of a program. For this reason, they may "forget" to make referrals, even when a particular family can afford the fees.

Overview of Research and Policy Issues

Research Issues

Research on respite and adult day care, especially in rural areas, is still in its infancy; therefore, results of studies conducted to date should be considered preliminary. Most studies have used small, unrepresentative samples, have lacked control groups, and have assessed only the short-term impact of programs. Control groups, when used, frequently have been inadequate; in some cases, control group members have used programs in quantities similar to treatment group members (Zarit, 1992).

Most studies have focused on urban programs and populations. Research is needed to document innovative and successful methods of service outreach and delivery to rural populations. The rural population is composed of diverse racial, ethnic, and religious groups, with distinct cultures and beliefs, yet very little is known about how to plan and deliver effective programs to ethnic minority families (*Multicultural Respite*, 1992).

Research is needed to identify more clearly the benefits of respite and adult day care for caregivers in rural areas. Reducing caregiver stress and enhancing caregiver well-being are primary purposes of respite programs. However, studies have yielded contradictory results. Although some studies have found that caregivers experienced improved physical and mental well-being, renewed confidence in their ability to continue as caregivers, and reduction of both subjective and objective burden as a result of respite (Montgomery & Borgatta, 1989; Sharlach & Frenzel, 1986), other studies have found no significant effects of respite on caregiver burden or mental health (Lawton, Brody, & Saperstein, 1989a, 1989b).

All caregivers are not alike. Therefore, their responses to any intervention are likely to differ. Although it is generally assumed that respite and adult day care are inherently beneficial to caregivers, the reasons a caregiver uses respite and day care, and how he or she spends time while using a program, may have an impact on how effective it is in alleviating stress (Lawton et al., 1989a; Montgomery & Borgatta, 1989; Wright, Lund, & Caserta, 1990). To determine the effectiveness of a medication, questions such as these are asked: For whom is the medication most appropriate? What is the needed therapeutic dose? Under what conditions is it most effective? How much is needed for how long for it to be most effective? For whom is it not as effective? Perhaps similar questions need to be addressed relative to respite and adult day care programs:

- In what situations and for whom are various types of respite most appropriate?
- Which caregivers benefit the most from respite and adult day care services? Why and in what ways do they benefit?
- Are there strategies that can maximize the potential benefits of respite and day care for caregivers?
- Are there situational factors—such as caregiver history, quality of caregiver-care receiver relationship, or history of caregiving—that influence a caregiver's response to respite and adult day care?
- How do cultural issues affect a caregiver's use of and response to respite and adult day care programs?

The role of respite and adult day care in a caregiver's decision to continue with or initiate caregiving also is not clear. According to Berry et al. (1991), "It is possible that those caregivers who are willing to provide care seek respite, instead of respite affecting one's decision to continue care or begin providing care" (p. 834). Controlled studies comparing users and nonusers of respite care are needed to answer this question.

Research is needed that focuses on the range of outcomes of respite and day care for the care receiver, as well as the caregiver, in rural areas. Outcome measures are also needed that are more sensitive to change. Most research on outcomes relative to the care receiver has focused on whether or not adult day care and respite programs delay or prevent institutionalization. However, whether respite or adult day care does or does not postpone institutionalization is still open to question (Callahan, 1989).

Policy and Practice Implications

In their review of interventions and strategies for family caregivers, Zarit and Teri (1991) assert that it is too early to draw conclusions from research in regard to clear directions for public policy. Based on the findings to date, however, we make the following recommendations in regard to policy and service delivery.

Include the caregiver in the client base. A family-oriented approach is needed in the development of policies and the provision of services in rural areas. Traditionally, however, the service delivery system has targeted the needs of frail older persons and largely neglected their caregivers. In part, this is because most funding has been limited to services provided directly to older persons. It is equally important to consider caregivers as clients, because when a caregiver's health and well-being deteriorate, the person to whom care is provided is also affected.

Develop a funding base. Programs often have failed because they did not have adequate funding. If respite and adult day care programs are to be viable in rural areas, greater financial assistance and a consistent funding base is needed (Lawton et al., 1989a). A subsidy may be critical in the development phase of a program (Rosenheimer & Francis, 1992). Currently, reimbursement is minimal or nonexistent in most cases. This lack of Medicare payment and third-party reimbursement has limited the development of respite and adult day care (Van Werkhooven, 1991-1992). Many health care professionals believe that the only solution is to include coverage for adult day care and respite care in any future health care financing reforms.

Give priority to in-home respite and services. The sparse population base in rural areas, the geographic separation of need and service, the difficulties families report in transporting relatives to programs outside of the home, and family preferences for in-home care (Brody et al., 1989; Lawton et al., 1989a, 1989b) all suggest that a high priority should be given to in-home programs. Although many rural areas support viable adult day care centers, congregate programs may not be the most appropriate or viable in others. The more rural an area, the more emphasis needs to be given to bringing the services to the people. In addition, rather than developing new programs, it may be better to consider how services currently available to the elderly can be adapted to address the needs of caregivers.

Provide financial support to families. When families provide care to frail and dependent older persons, significant savings result to society. According to Deimling (1989), respite services, if used as a preventive measure, may enable families to continue providing care for longer periods of time, even if the older persons become more dependent. However, the cost of services is a significant factor in accessibility for some rural families.

Meltzer (1982) recommends giving consideration to extending eligibility for respite services beyond state Medicaid eligibility levels, perhaps with sliding fee scales adjusted for income. One issue to be resolved is whose income should be used in determining eligibility when subsidy funds are available (Miller & Goldman, 1989)—the caregiver's, the care recipient's, or both?

Policy makers often fear that requests for services will be overwhelming if respite and adult day care are subsidized; yet studies show that caregivers, in general, are willing to pay what they can afford and are modest in their use of services (Brody et al., 1989; Henry, 1992; Meltzer, 1982). The fear of a woodwork effect—that is, that people will "come out of the woodwork" to use a service and overload the system if a service is made readily available—is not supported by research on respite and adult day care.

It is important that policy and practice also reflect the realities of rural America and not be based on myths, such as that formal services are less needed in rural areas because the family is stronger and better able to provide assistance or that all rural areas are the same geographically and ethnically. A program successful in one rural community may not be successful in another. Sensitivity to diversity is as important in rural as in urban America. Responding to the needs of elders and caregivers and developing the most appropriate programs requires an understanding of the uniqueness of each subculture—the role of elders, the family's role in providing care, health practices, beliefs about the aging process, and attitudes toward the use of services.

Summary and Conclusions

Respite and adult day care are important in the continuum of long-term care because of their role in supporting families who provide care to physically frail and mentally impaired older adults. A variety of approaches to providing respite and adult day care have developed, each with its own advantages and disadvantages. A combination of these approaches has the best chance of meeting the diverse needs of caregivers. For example, both emergency and planned respite care are necessary for the delivery of comprehensive services. For working caregivers, adult day care may be a priority. However, in rural areas it is generally not possible to provide a full range of such services. Therefore, it is critical to identify the priority service needs of caregivers in an area and how these needs can best be met cost-effectively.

Although respite and adult day care appear to be significant in sustaining the at-home caregiver, the development of programs has been limited, particularly in rural areas. Low population density often means there is not a sufficient number of clients to have a funding base for staff, facilities, and services. The lack of third-party reimbursement and the particular characteristics of the rural environment are two more factors limiting the development of programs.

The need for respite and adult day care can be expected to grow as the elderly population increases in size. However, establishing a respite or adult day care program is not easy, and building one takes time. It is unrealistic to expect that if a program is developed, people will just come. Start-up is usually slow, and extensive marketing is required to sell a program to both family caregivers and referral sources.

Continued research is needed to determine the efficacy of respite and adult day care. Information is needed on how caregivers who actively seek out formal respite and day care may differ from caregivers in general. The diversity among caregiving situations, service needs, and delivery approaches should be strongly considered in regard to program impact.

PART IV

Health Promotion and Care

This section includes four chapters that focus on improving the health and meeting the health care needs of rural older persons. In Chapter 9, Mockenhaupt and Muchow begin by noting that rural elderly health promotion and disease prevention services should be given much more attention than they currently receive, because research has shown that rural elders, in general, experience a high prevalence of chronic disability and have fewer health services and professionals available to them than are found in urban areas. Mockenhaupt and Muchow devote considerable space to an excellent practice-oriented review of program ideas and strategies for overcoming existing barriers. They note the importance of ensuring that programs are consistent with the values, behaviors, and needs of local rural populations and utilize a variety of local networks to disseminate program materials. They discuss specific strategies that help ensure success, such as coalition building, use of peer educators, church-based care, and self-care. As for salient policy issues, Mockenhaupt and Muchow argue that funding and insurance reimbursement for health promotion and disease prevention services must be increased if these services are to become more available to the rural elderly. Research on the relationships among risk factors, disease status, functional limitations, and disabilities in older rural populations is needed, as are evaluation studies of alternative health promotion and disease prevention strategies. They conclude that policy changes and additional research are needed if strategies aimed at improving the health knowledge and behaviors of rural elders are to become more effective.

In Chapter 10, Ralston and Cohen examine nutrition, a topic often given scant attention in studies of the health status of older rural persons. Although existing stereotypes support the notion that rural persons eat well because they live "close to the land," Ralston and Cohen begin by noting that rural elders are likely to have greater risk of poor nutritional status than are their urban counterparts. This is because they generally are older, have lower levels of income and education, and have fewer health and nutrition services available to them than do urban elders. Ralston and Cohen provide a detailed review of the existing literature, limited as it is, on the diet and nutritional status of the rural elderly. They then discuss the different aspects of rural living that contribute significantly to observed nutritional deficits, including rural values, attitudes toward economic status, access to food, and beliefs about food preparation, quality, and nutritional adequacy. They present an in-depth examination of the two major approaches generally used to improve the nutritional status of the elderly: using nutrition specialists or peer educators to provide nutrition information and education to change food choice and consumption patterns, and a variety of feeding programs (e.g., congregate, in-home, homemaker) designed to provide meals that meet minimum daily nutritional requirements. They also explore responses to some of the major challenges involved in providing nutritional services to rural elders, such as high-risk populations, food "values," access to food, and lack of services. Ralston and Cohen conclude with a consideration of major policy and research issues. They note that nutrition policy must be seen within the context of the declining fortunes of rural America over the past two decades. They express concern that many programs (including nutrition programs) are not adequately targeted to those in greatest need, and that the problems of rural elders are not adequately recognized. Finally, they argue that good rural nutrition policy requires much greater attention to conducting research on the nutritional status of rural elders and the effectiveness of alternative nutrition-related education and feeding programs.

Chapter 11, by Redford and Severns, examines the broad topic of in-home health care, which includes both "medical" and "social" services. The authors argue that the demographics of rural areas and generally disadvantaged health status of rural elders suggest considerable need for home health services. They provide a succinct review of a number of programs that traditionally provide home health care, including Medicare, Medicaid, Title XX of Social Security, Title III of the Older Americans Act, and Veterans Administration and state programs, and discuss examples of alternative funding approaches, such as social /health maintenance organizations, On-Lok, and state and local models. They also detail a number of community approaches to developing and integrating health and social in-home care that emphasize centralizing, diversifying, and coordinating services. Redford and Severns then present an insightful discussion of a number of problems generally encountered in developing and providing home care services in rural areas, including the physical environment, financing of care, rural population diversity, attitudes and values, and labor force availability and adequacy. They argue that a number of pieces must be put into place if a coordinated and comprehensive system of rural home health services is to become a reality. These include service planning based on standardized assessment, client follow-up and service plan revision, a client-provider relationship, quality assurance, integration of chronic and acute services, adequately and appropriately trained staff, adequate salaries for staff, financial viability, and leadership. Finally, they identify areas in which further research is needed.

The final chapter in Part IV is coauthored by Bane, Rathbone-McCuan, and Galliher. Of all the service needs of the rural elderly, perhaps less is known about and fewer services are available for mental health than any other. Consequently, this chapter takes a somewhat different tack than the others, presenting original research findings on the provision of mental health services as well as an analysis of program needs and approaches. The authors begin with a review of some of the environmental factors related to rural mental health problems. They note that very little is known about the prevalence of these problems for the rural elderly, partly because so few services are available to identify and treat them. Yet, the need for such services is probably at least as great as it is among the urban elderly. Bane et al. then move to an excellent examination of the availability, accessibility, and acceptability of mental health services in rural areas, pointing out the dearth of mental health professionals and hospital- and outpatient-based services. Indeed, they suggest that the capacity of rural community mental health centers to serve the elderly actually diminished in the 1980s, even as rural areas experienced an increased need for these services because of broad economic and social stresses. Bane and her colleagues also discuss various state- and local-level approaches to developing and providing mental health services to older rural populations. They describe specific mental health programs from several largely rural states and report findings from a recent survey of the need, availability, and funding of mental health services as reported by more than 400 Area Agencies on Aging. They conclude that mental health programs for the rural elderly should be integrated into social and health care planning, delivery, and financing systems in addition to being provided in more specialized psychiatric and mental health care areas.

9

Disease and Disability Prevention and Health Promotion for Rural Elders

ROBIN E. MOCKENHAUPT
JENNIFER A. MUCHOW

Services for disease and disability prevention and health promotion are some of the most important means of achieving good health and quality of life for older persons, allowing functional independence and aging in place. Although this holds true for rural, suburban, and urban elders, considerable barriers exist to the provision and availability of these essential services in rural communities. This is unfortunate for several reasons. Although rural and urban elders generally experience similar kinds of health problems, rural elders tend to be in poorer health than their urban counterparts on several indicators, especially in rates of chronic disease and disability. A large percentage of elderly persons living in nonmetropolitan areas assess their health as fair or poor (U.S. Senate, Special Committee on Aging, 1992). In addition, lack of economic resources and poverty among rural elders compound the situation; poverty negatively affects health, and ill health impoverishes. This chapter examines programmatic responses and strategies for overcoming barriers to the provision of services and programs aimed at disease and disability prevention and health promotion for rural elders. Some successful strategies that have been utilized in rural communities include coalition building, use of peer educators and volunteers, provision of services through religious institutions, and self-care. However, these strategies are found only in selected areas of the United States; more services and programs are needed in most rural communities. Later in this chapter we present an examination of research and policy issues in this area, as well as some recommendations for future programming.

Health Promotion, Disease Prevention, and Disability Prevention

Demographic, epidemiological, economic, and social changes among the older population have spurred the development of health promotion and disease and disability prevention programs to enhance healthy aging and improve quality of life for older persons. *Health promotion* for older adults has been defined as "planned action to maintain or improve physical, mental or spiritual health. It can be accomplished through personal or collective behavioral and environmental change. The best methods are those that promote dignity and independence, and build knowledge and skills to help older adults make informed, healthy choices, for themselves and their communities" (FallCreek, 1992, p. 5). Health promotion strategies are those related to individual lifestyle that can have a significant impact on a person's current and future health by preventing or minimizing the impact of disease (U.S. Department of Health and Human Services, 1990). These issues include physical activity and fitness, healthy nutrition, cessation of tobacco use, moderate use of alcohol, proper use of medications, mental health, injury prevention, oral health, and so on.

Disease prevention strategies for the early detection of disease include counseling, health screening, immunization, and the use of drugs to reduce the risk of developing a disease (Preventive Services Task Force, 1989). These strategies are most often provided in a clinical setting (i.e., a physician's office, hospital, or health clinic), but also can be provided in alternative settings, such as health fairs. *Disability prevention* strategies help older persons to manage existing chronic conditions so that they can function with maximum independence. Although most persons aged 65 and older have one or more chronic diseases (American Association of Retired Persons, 1991a), not all restrict their daily activities or functioning. Difficulty in performing daily tasks such as bathing, eating, or dressing leads to the need for assistance and often limits opportunities for elders to remain independent in the community

(U.S. Department of Health and Human Services, 1990). Disability prevention activities can help older persons remain independent and can extend years of "healthy life."

Health of Rural Elders

Research conducted with rural elders shows that it is difficult to identify geography as the leading risk factor for poor health status and as the cause of differences between rural and suburban or urban elders (Dwyer, Lee, & Coward, 1990; Lubben, Weiler, Chi, & De Jong, 1988). In addition, rural elders are a heterogeneous group, and their health status may be more influenced by characteristics other than rural residence, such as marital status, age, income, education, and race. However, as noted above, although rural and urban elders generally experience similar kinds of health problems, rural elders tend to be in poorer health than their urban counterparts on some indicators. Despite "within rural" (e.g., farm/nonfarm) distinctions in health status and self-perception of health, rural elders in general have "a relatively high prevalence of chronic disability and fatal injuries, combined with a lower prevalence of some key preventive behaviors (such as seat belt use)" (Office of Technology Assessment, 1990, p. 54). The disabilities are results of higher rates of chronic disease, such as arthritis, cardiovascular disease, hypertension, and diabetes (Coward & Dwyer, 1991a). Some studies also show that older rural adults do not regularly use positive health practices (Johnson, 1991; U.S. Senate, Special Committee on Aging, 1992). The Office of Technology Assessment (1990) suggests that "preventive and therapeutic health programs addressing these areas might be particularly appropriate to rural populations" (p. 54).

A major factor influencing health status, of course, is poverty. Although some retirement communities in rural America are thriving, there continues to be persistent poverty, especially in the South. Poverty is associated with poorer health among older persons and with the decreased use of health services (Coward & Dwyer, 1991a). Rural residents, including rural elders, have lower average incomes and higher poverty rates than do urban residents, and have fewer contacts with physicians and hospitals (Office of Technology Assessment, 1990). As hospitals and physicians are a source of health promotion and disease prevention programs, services, and information, an impoverished older person is both less likely to know of programs and less likely to be able to pay for health promotion or disease and disability prevention services. Although most rural elders are covered by Medicare (less than 1% lack any health insurance), they are less likely to have private insurance. Far too few preventive services are covered by any insurance program, public or private. This, combined with fewer resources for health promotion and disease prevention in the rural community, makes programs unavailable or financially inaccessible to rural elders.

Another factor that sometimes binds rural elders to poor health status is the characteristic of race or ethnicity. Although overall a higher proportion of white elders reside in rural communities, in some parts of the country rural populations comprise significant numbers of elders in particular racial or ethnic groups, for example, African American elders in the South and Hispanic elders in the Southwest and West. Many other minority groups also contribute to the rural melting pot. Given that minority members experience poorer health status and reduced utilization of health services, a rural-dwelling minority elder is at high risk for poor health as well as poverty. Being rural, poor, and elderly is sometimes called triple jeopardy. Add minority status to this combination and it become quadruple jeopardy. Too often in the past health promotion and disease prevention have been offered through mainstream networks and institutions, where minority elders were less likely to feel comfortable or welcome.

Rural elders as a group are clearly at high risk for poor health and disability. Understanding the characteristics, attitudes, and behaviors that put them at risk enables providers to plan health promotion programs and older persons to make changes in behavior to live healthier lives. However, the impact of "rurality" on the health and quality of lives of individuals in communities is defined locally, by examining geography, economics, current service provision, ethnicity, behaviors, and actual health status of individuals. Improved health status and quality of life can be realized through health promotion and disease and disability prevention, but barriers in a variety of guises must be recognized and overcome before all rural elders can benefit from the preventive model.

Service Provision and Utilization:
Barriers and Resources

Several authors have identified factors that can act as barriers to the provision and utilization of services and programs to rural elders (e.g.,

Bull, Howard, & Bane, 1991; Krout, 1988a). These challenges range from physical to political. Following are some examples of the ways in which health promotion and disease and disability prevention services are affected. Service providers may not be able to move mountains to make their programs more accessible, but creative ideas and continued effective advocacy can turn these challenges into opportunities for innovative programs, health care reform, and healthier older persons.

Physical Barriers

The isolation, distance, and transportation problems characteristic of rural areas create very apparent physical barriers to traditional methods of delivering health promotion messages and programs. Fortunately, health promotion messages actually lend themselves to a variety of delivery modes and messengers. Covering distances via the airways of radio and television, for instance, or hitching a ride with the letter carrier in a utility bill, are means of reaching older persons with health information and education. "Mail-order" health promotion interventions are being tested with older retirees in some California communities (Leigh et al., 1992). Not all rural elders have telephone service, but many do, and might use a health hot line. Groups of older persons can sometimes be reached in non-health care settings, where they may already be congregating for different purposes, such as at church or at a congregate meal site. In addition, self-care, an important part of some health promotion programs, is ideally suited to the geographic realities of rural life. There is accumulating evidence that effective at-home or self-management of chronic disease has a major positive impact on physical and psychological health status (Clark et al., 1991). Thus individuals need not lack information because of physical barriers alone.

For actual services, an obvious way to cope with physical barriers of distance, terrain, and lack of transportation is to "go to the people." However, public health nurses are limited in the numbers of visits they can make when clients live many miles apart. Meals on Wheels volunteers have to travel the same poorly maintained roads and cross the same bridges older persons would have to travel if they were to go to town for a meal at the senior center. Mobile health units have been used in some areas to provide some preventive services more commonly found in clinical settings, but quality and maintenance of equipment (e.g., X-ray machines) may be difficult to control. When physical barriers must be broken, not just bypassed, Bull et al. (1991) recommend advocacy by and alliances among those who share common needs and concerns, such as better transportation, roads, equipment, and personnel.

Economic Barriers

Poverty is widespread among rural elders, and with the cost of health care rising rapidly in recent years, economic barriers can outweigh even physical barriers. Rural elders are somewhat more likely than their urban counterparts to rely on Medicaid or other public programs, and are less likely to have private insurance to supplement Medicare coverage (Office of Technology Assessment, 1990). However, the real issue is that few health promotion and disease and disability prevention services are covered by any of these insurance programs. The traditional medical model of coverage for acute care is still promoted over the preventive model of coverage for a comprehensive array of disease prevention and health promotion services. Until there is widespread reimbursement for preventive care, all low-income groups will have limited access to preventive health services and programs.

Another economic barrier is frequently the poverty of the economy itself. In rural economies there may be few, if any, private funders for health promotion and disease prevention programs. In addition, where there is a rural hospital offering health promotion, the service is often viewed by the struggling hospital as an unnecessary luxury, and that service will often be the first cut in a financial crisis. Rural elders tend to receive fewer comprehensive health promotion services than do semi-rural or urban elders, according to a study of the California Preventive Health Care for the Aging Program (PHCAP) (Lubben et al., 1988). For instance, participants in the PHCAP sites were less likely to have received an annual examination than were other persons in the study.

In a poor economy even aging and health organizations may view health promotion as a luxury, reasoning that other institutions of the community will offer this service to elders. There can be successful wellness programs in rural hospitals, as described in a report produced by the American Hospital Association (Kernaghan, 1992), but they have relied on "a patchwork of financial support, in-kind contributions, and local donations" to support their efforts (p. 35). They reached out to other organizations in the community and found resources available.

Lack of Awareness

The distance and isolation of rural areas may result in a lack of awareness of services that do exist. One study found that residence in a small community or rural area was associated with awareness of fewer services (Krout, 1988a). This may indicate that rural providers are not aware of effective strategies for promoting programs, including publicity. Low literacy rates among rural elders and poorly designed materials (e.g., type size and style or poor contrast of paper and ink color) also may contribute to a lack of awareness of services that have been advertised. Professionals from formal health and aging networks must reach out to other networks, both formal and informal, such as religious institutions, community clubs, and volunteer groups, where personal contact will result in word-of-mouth communication.

Availability of Services

No national studies have been done of the availability of health promotion and disease and disability prevention programs and services for rural elders; the majority of research on programming that has been conducted has focused on urban elders (Johnson, 1991). Often rural elders are "handed scaled-down urban service models that fail to meet their needs or are insensitive to the real differences between urban and rural areas" (Van Hook, 1987). Traditional models of health promotion are delivered in urban areas through existing health and aging institutions. If fewer of these institutions (hospitals, clinics, physicians) exist in rural areas, then health promotion services are also offered to fewer older rural residents.

Attitudes

Aging stereotypes held by both older adults and service providers continue to be a major barrier to the provision and utilization of health promotion programs and services. "I'm too old to exercise" (or stop smoking, stop drinking, change my habits) is a common rationale given for not making lifestyle changes necessary to reduce risk for disease and disability. Rural elders and professionals maintain these attitudes, as their suburban and urban counterparts also do. This could be overcome, in part, by support for and adoption of a preventive model of health care in the United States. Young persons still grow up believing that disease is to be cured, not prevented, and that aging inevitably leads to disease and disability. Providers can help older persons experience short-term, as well as long-term, benefits from changing high-risk behaviors. Linking healthy behaviors with community and individual values, such as independence and thrift, can help to increase the value of health promotion in an older person's life.

Another potential attitude barrier is cultural insensitivity. Older adults and key leaders from the community should be an integral part of the planning and development of health promotion programs and services, and this is especially true if planners and target audiences differ in racial or ethnic backgrounds. Planners should educate themselves about traditional diets, folk remedies, and health beliefs and values. The psychological components of healing and staying healthy may be culture bound. Inclusion of traditional healers and respect for "old ways" will increase acceptance and credibility of health promotion and disease prevention services among elders. For example, among Native Americans, use of the "sweat lodge" is a common purification ceremony. As part of a health initiative funded by the Robert Wood Johnson Foundation, a 61-year-old Native American is bringing the concept of the sweat lodge to recovering alcoholics and drug addicts ("Native Americans Use," 1991). Another example is a health promotion/self-care effort targeted to Native American, Hispanic, and rural elders in New Mexico. A *curandera* (traditional folk healer) was added to the program in Hispanic communities to make the section on medication more relevant for the elders (Glassheim, n.d.).

Program Ideas and Strategies

Health promotion and disease prevention targeting of rural elders—that is, labeling and "publicizing" of rural elders as a high-risk group—is in itself unlikely to produce large changes in behavior in this population. Individuals who are labeled "high risk" are no more likely to change behaviors than are those labeled "low risk." Additionally, if rural elders are singled out from among all older adults for interventions, a large number of elders in the general population with similar but unidentified risk characteristics will be missed by the targeting and subsequent intervention efforts. Targeting can, however, draw attention to the needs of rural elders, and that attention is valuable if it initiates policy action and financial support favorable to rural areas.

Even without targeting, and despite barriers, rural elders have been and can continue to be reached with health promotion and disease and disability prevention programs. To reduce high-risk behaviors across the rural elderly population, however, it is imperative to tailor health promotion programs to the values and needs of small and rural communities based on knowledge of regional and economic differences. Because tailoring is more critical than targeting for purposes of behavior change, health promotion is and should continue to be delivered to rural elders through a variety of networks. These include cooperative extension, public health departments, hospitals, Area Agencies on Aging, local-level senior centers, colleges and universities, and community service agencies, such as mental health centers. Churches, long recognized as important vehicles for information in many rural areas, have recently begun to offer more health-specific information and monitoring of congregations. The structure, mission, and resources of each of these networks have determined the programming approach taken. With the exception of some public health initiatives, however, there is too often little community-based planning involved in these efforts.

Although there are always examples to hold up (sometimes for political purposes) of programs "run on a shoestring," the costs of programming can be discouraging to even the most dedicated coordinator, who must budget for such expenses as how-to manuals, long-distance phone calls for advice ("technical assistance"), transportation, staff, facilities, snacks, equipment, and publicity. A well-established service, such as a meal program, may be written into the budget year after year. Public health nurses continue to be funded to reach out to rural underserved elders as well as to those of all other ages. Unfortunately, however, many health promotion and disease and disability prevention interventions do not have a long history in rural areas—or any history at all. Advocating for a piece of the diminishing budget pie is usually easier for those who clearly see and believe in the ability of health promotion programs to enhance elders' lives.

Several strategies can be identified that successfully overcome at least some of the barriers to health promotion in rural areas. One enthusiastic and persistent individual who can "carry" a program until it has had time to prove itself successful can be critical. Some of the strategies and examples of programs described in this section are quite flexible and lend themselves to a variety of sponsoring groups and communities; others need certain supportive resources that will not be available in all communities. The program examples are meant to bring the strategies to life, as well as to inspire others to think about how these ideas might be adapted to their own communities of elders. A list of the programs mentioned, with contact information, is provided in the appendix to this chapter.

Coalition Building

The 1990s are the decade of coalition building. Competition is out, or should be, in rural areas. With a shortage of financial and human resources and a health service infrastructure that can collapse like a house of cards if the local hospital closes, rural practitioners serving elders must choose partners wisely, but choose them they must.

Coalitions take a variety of forms, and may be undertaken for many reasons. For example, individuals from different agencies might wish to work together informally to share information or expertise. More formally, organizations sometimes find it mutually beneficial to link up temporarily to achieve a short-term goal, perhaps through a subcontract or "letter of agreement." Of course, any partner who can provide even partial funding for a program will be much sought after. Although the relative deprivation of rural economies includes a lack of private and corporate philanthropies, the value to businesses—in terms of goodwill as well as marketing—of an agency's access to older adults is often overlooked.

Rural hospitals joining with their communities to solve mutual problems are using coalition building to increase residents' loyalty to the institution and to decrease the problem of underutilization, a contributing factor in hospital closure. As a report released by the American Hospital Association points out, "Health promotion is a useful medium for forging strong community linkages—for enhancing community-hospital relations, for initiating a forum for local health planning, and for developing collaborative efforts with other community providers and agencies" (Kernaghan, 1992, pp. 33-34). The report also offers a "list of essential ingredients to successful community health promotion" as described by hospitals that have done it, including, "Erase all arbitrary barriers both in terms of what the coalition can do and who can do it" (p. 35).

Another kind of alliance can involve non-health care businesses or corporations whose customers include older adults. The Gatekeeper Training Program, part of the Elderly Outreach Services of the Abbe Center for Community Mental Health in Cedar Rapids, Iowa, is just such an alliance. A rural version of the Gatekeeper Training Program at the Spokane Community Mental Health Center in Washington, the Iowa program addresses several of the major barriers to rural mental health promotion and disease prevention.

The concept of the Gatekeeper Program is to train community workers who, through their regular business activities, come in contact with elderly people. These workers, or gatekeepers, may include utility repair personnel, meter readers, postal workers, bank personnel, fuel oil dealers, and others. The gatekeepers are trained to recognize early changes in the activities, behaviors, habits, or conversation of elders that might indicate mental problems and then to take steps to ensure that at-risk elders get help.

Although urban elders living alone can be isolated, too, confined by fear of crime as well as frail health, the geographic conditions, compounded by low population size and density, that isolate many rural elders living alone put them at particular risk and make identifying them even more problematic for mental health professionals. These older adults may not recognize their own cognitive impairment or may not seek help because of their desire for independence or suspicion of mental health services. Identifying and monitoring at-risk isolated elders may easily require more resources in time, transportation, and personnel than one rural agency can provide, particularly if it is serving a large region. With the cooperation of trained gatekeepers, however, significantly more of these individuals may benefit from early interventions when the appropriate referral is made.

Peer Educators

Lack of a trained labor pool for delivering rural health promotion programs may be one reason for using peer educators, but those who have successfully employed this strategy will say it is not the only or even the best reason. Trained older adults from the community can offer a bridge over the barrier of cultural differences that may exist, particularly in the very independent old-old rural cohort or in minority elders who have suffered institutionalized racism and whose values, beliefs, and even language may differ from the mainstream. Studies also indicate that peer leader programs are an effective way to reach low socioeconomic status groups (Kottke, 1986). The peer educators themselves increase their health knowledge and sometimes their self-esteem and leadership capabilities as a result of their training and experience.

Peer educators deliver their health messages using various formats. Trained "volunteer visitors" actually go into the homes of frail elders as part of the South Santee Community Center's Homebound Support Program in McClellanville, South Carolina. They address home safety, nutrition, and physical activity issues and at the same time provide companionship to this sometimes neglected group of people. The volunteers' one-on-one instruction helps overcome the problem of low literacy rates among rural elders. These peer educators have essentially become part of a case management effort, identifying needs to which resources can then be matched.

Another way to overcome the low literacy problem is by using videotapes. The Minority Peer Educator Program at the Texas Agricultural Extension Service in College Station has put an entertaining "soap opera" with a strong health message for older adults together with peer educators to lead a discussion following the show. In reality four separate programs, two targeting black elders and two Hispanic elders, the Minority Peer Educator Program was developed for use at senior nutrition sites. Each videotape tackles a specific health problem, for example, high blood pressure in black elders. Actors create a realistic scenario, incorporating health information and addressing myths and misinformation. Trained peer educators, with whom the audience can identify, provide the personal follow-up needed for encouraging lifestyle changes.

Bringing health promotion to locations where rural elders already congregate, such as nutrition/meal sites, overcomes the barrier that transportation so frequently poses. Not all older adults gather in one particular place, of course, or at one particular time. Priorities have to be set and plans for programs made based on a combination of need, budget, and staffing. The two programs described briefly above show how peer educators can be used to reach older adults in different circumstances. The older adults to be reached also determine those who may be trained as peer educators. An older adult who is not a true peer of the audience may seem "out of context," whether that context is socioeconomic, racial, cultural, or educational.

When needs are great, it is difficult to make choices regarding whose needs should be met. Frail, homebound elders are often in dire need of assistance, especially if they are geographically isolated by terrain or distance and living alone. However, fewer of these at-risk elders can be reached—only as many as there are volunteers (who may have transportation difficulties of their own). Seniors who are able to come to a meal site may not be as imminently at risk, but certainly more of them can be reached with the same resources, and they are equally deserving of programs. There is no good answer to this dilemma. Rural practitioners and residents have often "made do" with less than their urban counterparts and have learned to work through informal networks. Unfortunately, this circumstance has sometimes been used to rationalize the withholding of formal supports and services.

Church-Based Health Promotion

Health promotion and disease and disability prevention services are beginning to be delivered in a deliberate and successful way through religious communities. Churches are often "insiders" in rural areas, where outsiders may be viewed with suspicion. For rural minority elders, the church may represent the community institution of greatest familiarity and acceptance. This does not mean, however, that an individual of one denomination will visit a church of another denomination to take advantage of a health education or health screening program. Church-based health promotion is most successful when it takes place within congregations and is incorporated into the healing mission and hierarchy of church leadership.

The Parish Nurse Project out of the Northwest Aging Association in Spencer, Iowa, was so successful when initially funded in 1989 that additional funding was awarded by the W. K. Kellogg Foundation to expand the project. Parish nurses, who are registered nurses and supported by their parish and religious leaders, are involved in a variety of activities, including organizing health fairs, writing health articles for church newsletters, making presentations, providing blood pressure screenings, referring to community health and social service resources, making home visits, and coordinating support groups. Parish nurses are in churches with as few as 50 members to as many as 3,000. Their validation of the spiritual component of health and healing (holistic wellness) while emphasizing self-responsibility is an effective approach for many church-affiliated rural elders.

Church-based health promotion requires the support of clergy, whether the health programs are coordinated by nurses or lay volunteers. In some rural areas, such as parts of Appalachia, ministers traditionally travel from place to place, preaching to congregations that gather when word passes that the minister has arrived. Efforts by outside agencies to reach elders with health promotion programs through the church may be well-intentioned but futile under these circumstances. In other cases, however, church-agency collaborations are reasonable and realistic, provided agency staff know and respect the context in which health is understood by the particular religion.

Self-Care

Self-care as a strategy for health promotion and disease and disability prevention would seem to be a "natural" for rural elders. The common physical and economic barriers to health care in rural areas demand a self-reliance of residents that is often a source of great pride. However, self-care must be appropriate to be effective. As one study of self-care behaviors in a frontier area of Idaho revealed, self-medicating with both prescription and nonprescription medications was common (Bartlome, Bartlome, & Bradham, 1992). Because more than 20% of the study respondents used nonprescription medications inappropriately, the authors suggest that "educational interventions . . . may be effective in avoiding inappropriate or hazardous self-medication practices by rural and frontier residents" (p. 11). They also conclude that self-care practices may assist in cost containment and suggest that third-party payers "include considerations of self-care practices and illness behaviors of rural and frontier residents in their service planning" (p. 11).

Recognizing that 70-80% of health problems that older adults deal with are handled in the home, Healthwise, Inc., of Boise, Idaho, developed Healthwise for Life, a medical self-care education program consisting of a workshop and book. Collaborating with the Brookdale Foundation and the National Rural Health Network, Healthwise for Life has been used in rural areas with companies hoping to reduce retiree health care costs. Older adults leave the workshop with a clearly written reference book for practicing not only medical self-care at home, but good consumer skills when they do need to enter the formal medical care system. Emphasis is placed on recognition and appropriate management of symptoms, the right time to call a health professional, and active participation in the patient-doctor partnership.

Rural areas often possess a rich folklore of self-care instructions. "Granny's remedy" may or may not have a factual basis; what is important is the sense of control one maintains in its administration. The "new, improved" self-care maintains this control and seeks to extend it into the relationship the individual has with a health care provider. Whether the condition is chronic or acute, appropriate action at home may relieve discomfort and prevent or delay dangerous and costly medical crises. For a variety of reasons, physicians have not always looked favorably on medical self-care, but the time may be right for rural doctors in particular to embrace a more flexible model of the patient-doctor relationship. Physical barriers and health personnel shortages in rural areas all too often cause dangerous time delays in treatment. Provided they are convinced that the self-care is medically sound, physicians can and should be allies in this strategy.

Whereas the doctor's goal for medical self-care may be reducing the number of both unnecessary and crisis visits, the goal for businesses clearly is reducing costs associated with these types of health care utilization. Although evaluation research is currently incomplete for some self-care programs, one study has shown that participants saved $133 per person per year in medical costs, with doctor visits decreased by 7% and hospital days reduced by 27% (Harrington & Richardson, 1990). For rural elders, who are more likely to rely on Medicare and Medicaid and less likely to have private insurance than are urban elders, the savings accrue to the two government programs or to their own pockets.

Programming That Is Most Needed

The programming that is most needed and will bring the best results in rural areas is community based, tailored to the geographic region, and comprehensive. An important factor to consider in planning strategies with limited resources is whether to try to change one behavior known to be risky or several risky behaviors at once. The temptation might be to identify, through screening tests, all those elders at highest risk for a major disease and then target only this group for an intervention. This could be a costly mistake, however. As Kottke (1986) has pointed out, screening for the high-risk subpopulation "consumes funds that could be used for intervention and may give people false assurance that they can continue high-risk behaviors" (p. 31). That is, those who are not labeled "high risk" see themselves as having no risk. In addition, those who are high risk are no more likely to change behaviors following intervention than are those who are low risk.

If a practitioner is dealing with a population—say the elders of the entire county—an effective approach is to address many risk factors simultaneously. This approach will be more attractive to a greater number of people than will an intervention aimed at a single risk factor. It will result in smaller changes, but across multiple behaviors in a large number of people. If a practitioner is working with individuals—say a physician working to reduce heart disease risk in a patient who smokes—a single-factor intervention will be more effective and can result in a large behavior change for that specific behavior. In this circumstance the individual is already screened or self-screened. Of course, the intervention aimed at a single risk factor may include many different strategies, but all would attempt to change just one behavior.

In rural areas, where there are few people to begin with and they may be scattered geographically, there simply may not be the resources to provide interventions concerned with single risk factors, as these interventions will generally attract fewer individuals and be less cost-effective. Both types of interventions are valuable, but an intervention designed to address multiple risk factors, tailored to the beliefs and values of specific communities, is likely to provide the greatest benefit overall for the least cost.

Research and Policy Issues

A primary barrier to the utilization of preventive services, and to the development and utilization of health promotion programs and services, is cost. For many adults, out-of-pocket payments are the primary source of funding for preventive services (such as screening for detection of disease) and other types of health promotion programs. Most private and public health insurance does not cover many health promotion or disease prevention services. For example, only four preventive services are currently covered under Medicare: pneumococcal vaccine, hepatitis B vaccine for high-risk individuals, pap smears every three years for women (or more frequently for women at high risk), and mammography screening for women aged 65 and older, every year for disabled women aged 50 to 64, every other year for women with disabilities aged 40 to 50, and every three years for disabled women aged 35 to 40. Original provisions in the Older Americans Act for the financing and delivery of preventive services have never been realized, owing to lack of appropriations for those services. Reimbursement for health promotion and disease prevention activities in rural areas is essential to the provision of services. Until adequately addressed through health care reform or through other legislative means, this will remain at the root of barriers to the provision and utilization of health promotion and disease and disability prevention services. In addition, research is needed to examine the reduction of financial barriers to care for rural older persons, particularly related to long-term care and rehabilitation (which include disability prevention services), mental health, disease prevention, and health promotion services.

A variety of health care providers, such as nurses and nurse practitioners, physician's assistants, social workers, health educators, occupational and physical therapists, and dietitians, should be licensed, utilized, and reimbursed for providing health promotion services to rural elders. In many areas with no physicians, these professionals are the only providers of medical and/or health care. They could be a valuable resource in the provision of health promotion and disease and disability prevention services in many rural areas. Nontraditional programs and providers of health promotion services, including non-health care paid or volunteer staff, also should be encouraged and supported, with special emphasis on utilization of innovative methods to reach and motivate rural elders.

The relationships among risk factors, disease conditions, health status, functional limitation, and disability need further research with older populations. Many lifestyle prescriptions are still based on research on younger populations. More research is needed that explores the relationship of demographic variables (e.g., geography, age, race) to the health status of rural elders. Clinical research into the causes, prevention, management, and rehabilitation of functional disability in older persons is vital, as functional disability is the major obstacle to independence in older persons (Institute of Medicine, 1991). Areas of exploration should include muscle strength and mobility, medication management, urinary incontinence, and fall-related injuries. Behavioral and social research should focus on the postponement of disability and dependence, particularly in women, minorities, and rural elders. Research is also needed to determine the efficacy and cost-effectiveness of health promotion and disease and disability prevention programs, and of alternative means of delivering them.

Once the need for intervention is supported, the attainment of good health for older persons will depend on educational and community-based interventions and programs to promote good health and prevent disease. These programs must attempt to reach individuals outside of traditional health care settings, which are sometimes scarce in rural areas. Research is needed to evaluate the impact of health education approaches on risk factors, morbidity, quality of life, and mortality, especially with special populations of rural elders.

Community-based programs may address a single risk factor or health problem, or may address several problems. A single activity or action may be initiated to encourage or support change, whereas a program with multiple interventions is often planned and coordinated by several agencies within the community. One of the Year 2000 Objectives for the Nation is to "increase to at least 90% the proportion of people aged 65 and older who had the opportunity to participate during the preceding year in at least one organized health promotion program through a senior center, lifecare facility, or other community-based setting that serves older adults" (U.S. Department of Health and Human Services, 1990, p. 257). Community-based programs may also include outreach activities designed for persons outside the setting and those most likely to be at high risk (e.g., homebound elders). In rural areas, new models are needed for delivering appropriate behavior change programs to older adults. Many variables have yet to be identified that promote or impede success in the practical application of research to programs. Finally, demonstration projects are needed to deliver preventive and health promotion services to older persons in rural areas.

Summary and Conclusions

Health promotion and disease and disability prevention can help older persons, including rural elders, stay independent as they age. Rural elders do experience higher rates of some chronic diseases, and have more medical conditions and functional limitations than their urban and suburban counterparts. Race and economic conditions also affect their health status. In addition, factors such as lack of transportation, poor accessibility of services, and cost of services can prove to be barriers to achieving good health status and quality of life.

To achieve good health status for rural elders, health promotion and disease and disability prevention programs need to be tailored to the values and needs of rural communities based on knowledge of regional and economic differences. A variety of networks can be used as delivery mechanisms, many of which exist in rural communities: churches, cooperative extension, public health departments, hospitals, and other community service agencies. Successful strategies to overcome the barriers presented by rural settings include coalition building, a mechanism for agencies to join together to solve mutual problems and achieve common goals; use of peer educators, trained older adults who lead programs on a number of health promotion topics; church-based health promotion, such as the parish nurse project described above, which emphasizes the holistic health philosophy of physical, emotional, and spiritual well-being; and use of self-care. Whether through interventions targeting single or multiple risk factors, increased quality of life can be achieved by offering health promotion and disease and disability prevention programs in rural communities. Legislative and policy changes at national and state levels must address the need for prevention activities in health care reform over the remaining years of the 1990s.

Appendix: Model Programs in Health Promotion

Gatekeeper Training Program
Abbe Center for Community Mental Health
520 Eleventh Street, N.W.
Cedar Rapids, IA 52405
(319) 398-3562

Homebound Support Program
South Santee Community Center
710 South Santee Road
McClellanville, SC 29458
(803) 546-2789

Minority Peer Educator Program
Texas Agricultural Extension Service
Texas A&M University
205C Special Services Building
College Station, TX 77843-2251
(409) 845-1146

Parish Nurse Project
Northwest Aging Association
2 Grand Avenue
Spencer, IA 51301-0310
(712) 262-1775

Healthwise for Life
Healthwise, Inc.
P.O. Box 1989
Boise, ID 83701
(208) 345-1161

10

Nutrition and the Rural Elderly

PENNY A. RALSTON
NANCY L. COHEN

Although diet and nutrition are critical for health promotion and disease prevention in persons of all ages, nutrition is especially important for maintaining independence and quality of life in the elderly. However, certain older populations, such as the rural elderly, may be at added risk with regard to nutritional status. There are fewer health services in rural areas compared with urban areas (Rogers, 1991), and rural elderly have higher health expenditures than do urban elders (Schwenk, 1992). Further, the rural elderly are older and have lower incomes and less education than urban elderly (Schwenk, 1992), and these demographic factors are related to poor nutritional outcomes (Guthrie, Black, & Madden, 1972; Norton & Wozny, 1984). Despite the potential for added nutritional risk in the rural elderly, information about the nutritional status of this group is sparse and sometimes conflicting (Calasanti & Hendricks, 1986; Norton & Wozny, 1984). Seniors residing in rural areas comprise a heterogeneous population (Coward, 1979), thus certain subgroups of this population may be at high risk for poor nutritional status and others may be at lower risk for certain nutrition-related problems.

We begin this chapter with a review of the need for nutritional services by the rural elderly, with focus on those subgroups of rural elderly who may have the greatest need. We then discuss the strategies that might serve as appropriate interventions in delivering nutritional services, examining both nutrition education and service delivery models. Finally, we highlight problems and needed programs for delivering nutritional services, along with research needs and policy issues.

The Nutrition Situation of the Rural Elderly

Diet is related to numerous risk factors for disability among the elderly, including high blood pressure, physical inactivity, polypharmacy, poor oral health, and osteoporosis (Berg & Cassels, 1990). Conversely, disease states prevalent in the elderly can influence the nutrient intake of this population. Atherosclerosis, cancer, dental decay, depression, diabetes, high blood pressure, osteoporosis, arthritis, and stroke can all lead to poor nutritional status (Berg & Cassels, 1990). Clearly, these risk factors and disease states are related to diet in both rural and urban elderly.

Research conducted on rural elderly populations shows low consumption of energy and calcium (Guthrie et al., 1972; Koh & Caples, 1979; Lee et al., 1991; Rawson, Weinberg, Herold, & Holtz, 1978). In contrast, rural elderly consume adequate levels of protein, iron, niacin, and vitamin C (Fosmire, Manuel, & Smiciklas-Wright, 1984; Koh & Caples, 1979; Lee et al., 1991; Rawson et al., 1978). Vitamin A intakes have been shown to be low (Guthrie et al., 1972; Rawson et al., 1978) or moderate (Lee et al., 1991) in this group. The average nutrient intakes of the rural elderly are similar to those of an urban population (Hollingsworth & Hart, 1991; Norton & Wozny, 1984; Stevens, Grivetti, & McDonald, 1992), but lower than those of a suburban population (Norton & Wozny, 1984). The difference in nutrient intakes between the rural and suburban populations has been attributed to differences in the education and income levels between these two groups (Norton & Wozny, 1984). Although, on average, the nutrient intakes of rural and urban elders are similar, the dietary intake of rural seniors varies with season more than does that of their urban counterparts. For example, Hollingsworth and Hart (1991) report that calcium intakes of rural elders are higher in the winter than in fall or summer.

Studies of intragroup differences within the rural elderly population are useful in revealing subgroups who are at potential nutritional risk. The older rural elderly consume fewer kilocalories than do younger rural seniors (Guthrie et al., 1972), with lower density of protein and niacin in the diet (Lee et al., 1991). Stevens et al. (1992) also report that older rural elders have poorer food choices than younger elders. On the other hand, carbohydrate and calcium intakes per 1,000 kilocalories are higher in older than in younger rural seniors (Lee et al., 1991).

Low income is also related to poor nutritional status in rural seniors. Learner and Kivett (1981) report that, among their sample, those rural elders with inadequate finances to meet their needs had lower self-perceived dietary adequacy than those with adequate finances. Low income has been related to decreased protein, iron, riboflavin, meat, and fruit intake in rural seniors (Guthrie et al., 1972). That study also showed that low-income rural elderly had lower education, poorer health status, increased chewing problems, and lower food expenditures than did their high-income peers.

Gender is another factor that is related to nutrition outcome in rural seniors. Rural elderly males, in comparison with females, have lower intakes of vitamin A (Koh & Caples, 1979; Rawson et al., 1978), niacin (Koh & Caples, 1979), and vitamin C (Hollingsworth & Hart, 1991). Research on the energy intakes of males and females is contradictory (Lee et al., 1991; Rawson et al., 1978) and may reflect differences in the specific populations studied.

With regard to race, several studies have shown that rural black elderly have poorer dietary quality than do rural white elderly. One study of an elderly population that included rural seniors showed that blacks had lower intakes of energy, protein, calcium, iron, and vitamin C than whites (Norton & Wozny, 1984). In addition, rural elderly blacks had a lower mean nutrient intake index (Lee et al., 1991) and lower self-reported dietary adequacy than whites (Learner & Kivett, 1981). Dietary adequacy was also related to low morale, poor self-rated health, and dissatisfaction with the frequency of visits with family and friends among the rural black elderly (Learner & Kivett, 1981).

In summary, the research regarding nutritional status of the rural elderly is sparse, but information that is available shows that their nutrient intake is similar to that of urban elderly. However, studies show that rural elderly consume less energy and calcium and have higher intakes of calcium in the winter months than do urban elderly. Rural elders who are older, male, and black and who have lower incomes are at greatest nutritional risk.

Factors Influencing Nutrition Among the Rural Elderly

There is a commonly held notion that "the rural environment" plays an indirect role in the nutritional well-being and general health of elderly living in rural areas. McCoy and Brown (1978) point out that "residential location represents experience over a period of time within a given life space—including the effects of environmental, economic, cultural and institutional forces" (p. 14). For elderly in rural areas, continuous rural residence includes unique life events that, socially and economically, have a cumulative effect on their lives (McCoy & Brown, 1978). Thus interconnected factors such as lower income, poorer health, inferior housing, and inadequate transportation, when sustained over time, provide a "rural effect" that goes beyond the sheer fact that the elderly person happens to reside in a rural area.

The rural environment is usually characterized by certain values and beliefs that can also have an impact on the nutrition of rural elderly. Krout (1986) points out that some of the values important to the lives of rural people include practicality, efficiency, work, friendliness, honesty, patriotism, deep religious commitment, social conservatism, and a mistrust of government. Rural people are often characterized as fiercely independent, and, coupled with their mistrust of the government, this results in lack of utilization of the few services that are available in rural areas. The values outlined above permeate the beliefs that rural people have toward food. Briley (1989) points out that previous eating habits play a large part in food selection of the elderly. For rural people, particularly those who were raised on farms, there may be certain beliefs about the preparation methods, quality, and nutritional adequacy of food that are based on earlier eating habits. Those beliefs may include the desire for "homemade" dishes that come from foods that have been raised in nearby gardens, with meals consumed in a warm family environment, as indicated in the following excerpt from the summary report of the National Strategy Conference on Improving Service Delivery to Rural Elderly:

> Portions are generous, three hearty meals a day are prepared, every item is "homemade" from scratch with no substitutions or preservatives, content may not be balanced but definitely contains a higher-than-required carbohydrate content, and eating is enjoyable family time in one's own home. (Farmers Home Administration, 1980, p. 22)

Clearly, rural elderly with this mental picture of a nutritious meal may have problems adjusting to congregate meals or other meal programs that, of necessity, may include institutional food preparation, limited portions, and less familiar people and surroundings (Farmers Home Administration, 1980).

In contrast to this perception of food, rural elders' attitudes toward their economic status are characterized as "making do," contributing to the tendency to cut food purchases to accommodate income limitations

(Glover, 1981; Heltsley, 1976). Moreover, when money is spent on food, it constitutes about a third of household expenditures (Lee et al., 1991). Although the need for help with food costs is apparent, rural elderly often do not seek assistance. Parks (1988), for example, reports that only 15% of the black rural elderly surveyed sought help in paying for food. Thus rural elderly not only frequently "make do," they also do not seek help with meeting their food needs.

Rural elderly find other problems in getting food. Transportation is a perennial problem in rural areas, but becomes even more of a critical issue for rural elders' acquisition of food items (Glover, 1981). Yearwood and Dressel (1983) report that congregate meal participants in rural areas must sometimes ride in vans or personal cars for 20 miles or more to reach a meal site. Hollingsworth and Hart (1991) report that, with increasing mobility problems, rural elderly may postpone shopping trips and delay restocking grocery items. Glover's (1981) study confirms that physical condition as well as transportation play important roles in rural elders' access to food. Among her sample, fatigue was the most common shopping problem, followed by transportation and difficulties in finding food.

Although acquisition of food is a perennial problem for rural elderly, social supports, both formal and informal, play a more positive role in the nutrition of rural elderly. With regard to formal supports, there is considerable evidence that rural elderly suffer distinct disadvantages in service delivery in comparison with urban elderly (Krout, 1986). However, certain food-related programs have grown in numbers in rural areas and are relatively prevalent in comparison with other services. Taietz and Milton (1979), for example, in their study of 53 upstate New York counties, report that between 1967 and 1976 services such as home health aides and home-delivered meals substantially increased more in rural counties than in urban counties. Nelson (1980) reports that, in a national sample of Area Agencies on Aging (AAAs), homemaker services (50%) and meals programs (34%) in rural AAAs were third and fifth in frequency, respectively, following transportation (93%) and information and referral (85%). In a more recent national study conducted in 1987, Krout (1989a) found that congregate and in-home meals were reported to be available by all of the AAA directors. Rural AAA directors placed these programs among the top five "most needed" services for the elderly in their areas.

Family, friends, and neighbors are also important in helping rural elderly maintain nutritionally adequate diets. Informal supports for rural elderly are similar to those of urban elderly, except that rural elderly (a) are more likely to live with their spouses, (b) have more male-headed households of two or more persons and fewer single women living alone, (c) have fewer children live in the same community but at least one child readily accessible, and (d) have more social contact with friends and neighbors (Mercier & Powers, 1984). Krout (1986) reports that the assistance that rural elders receive from informal supports is in nonpersonal areas, such as housework, shopping, and transportation, rather than in personal areas (e.g., dressing, bathing). It is in these nonpersonal areas where acquisition of food may be provided by the rural elder's social network. About 20-30% of the rural elderly receive help in meal preparation, and the majority of those providing help are family members or friends (Lee et al., 1991; Parks, 1988). In fact, Stevens et al. (1992) report that rural elderly rely on family for shopping and cooking assistance more than do urban elders. Also, not surprisingly, men more than women received help with meal preparation (Parks, 1988). Thus family, friends, and other informal members of the social network may be particularly important for adequate nutrition of rural elderly.

In summary, the nutrition of the rural elderly may be related to several factors. The rural environment is characterized by certain values, including beliefs about preparation methods, quality, and nutritional adequacy of food. Attitudes toward economic status, which are often characterized by conservative financial practices because of limited incomes, can also affect the amount of money rural elderly allocate toward food. Access to food is further complicated by transportation and other logistical problems, but rural areas do have formal food-related services available. The large majority of rural elderly shop for and prepare their own meals, but those who need help depend on family, friends, and neighbors.

Strategies for Intervention

There are two generally accepted strategies for improving the nutritional status of the elderly. One involves providing nutrition information in a variety of ways, including through nutrition specialists and peers, with the ultimate goal of changing food choice and food consumption behaviors. The second strategy involves direct provision of food through group feeding programs, home-delivered meals, homemaker services, and food stamps and other government-sponsored programs, with the overall goal of ensuring that the elderly's diets meet minimum daily nutritional requirements. Both of these models are examined below in light of their effectiveness in improving the nutritional status of the rural elderly.

Nutrition Education Models

There has been increased emphasis on nutrition education for elderly populations (Dwyer, 1980; Smiciklas-Wright, 1981), but limited research has been conducted related to the effectiveness of nutrition education models. For rural elderly populations, such research is almost nonexistent. Thus this discussion of nutrition education models will focus on general older adult populations, pointing out, where possible, studies on rural elderly.

Nutrition education that is delivered through use of nutrition specialists (broadly defined as those with nutrition expertise) can incorporate various educational methods. The most common method used is an ongoing series of lessons taught by the nutrition specialist. Colson and Green (1991) used an eight-week nutrition education program on sodium status and health to investigate changes in knowledge and status of selected minerals in 41 urban elderly subjects grouped into hypertension/control and normotensive/control groups. The findings showed that the program was somewhat effective in influencing dietary habits and very effective in increasing nutrition knowledge. There was more change in the hypertensive group than in the normotensive group, indicating that elderly with medical needs for dietary modification are most likely to change dietary habits and learn from nutrition education programs.

Williams, Kim, and McMullen (1986) developed nutrition lessons presented over an eight-week period intended to increase dietary intakes of calcium, magnesium, and potassium and to decrease sodium in a small sample of hypertensive elderly. An eight-week phase without nutrition education was included in the design to determine retention of nutrition lesson content. Dietary intake data using food recall procedures showed some changes in intakes for the four nutrients studied. However, blood serum levels of the nutrients did not significantly change in either the experimental or the control group during the study span. The authors conclude that nutrition education can be a positive influence on the dietary intakes of hypertensive elderly, and that dietary alterations may offer the most optimistic approach to lowering blood pressure levels of borderline hypertensive patients.

Wong, Krondl, and Williams (1982) determined the long-term effects of a nutrition intervention program for noninstitutionalized urban elderly in terms of maintenance and/or improvement of dietary practices. The intervention included use of 14 "marker" foods in discussions of nutrition and consumer issues, in food demonstrations, or in recipe distribution to participants. Foods were chosen for their nutrient content, the food groups they represented, their frequency of use, and their accessibility and price in the market. The design included pre- and posttest comparisons between the experimental group ($n = 56$) and a control group ($n = 50$) after the three-year project was completed. One of the striking features throughout the evaluation was the minimal but consistent positive change in program participants when compared with the control group. In general, greatest change was seen in knowledge of nutritive value of the marker foods (29%), followed by change in perception of food (18.2%) and change in food practices (7.7%). The authors conclude that the direct nutritional impact of the program was minimal, but that the study did document the continuous process of change in eating patterns of seniors.

The only study that has investigated nutrition education with a rural elderly population using the nutrition specialist model was conducted by Sorenson and Ford (1981). These researchers developed a one-day workshop to deliver practical information on the relationship of diet and health to older adults in senior centers in five rural areas in a western state. The workshop, which was taught by a team of professionals that included a family practitioner/gerontologist, a health educator, a nutrition specialist, and an extension specialist, had three major objectives: to help the elderly understand the role of obesity as a risk factor in chronic disease, to help elderly consumers identify their individual dietary goals, and to identify ways to help seniors achieve their dietary goals. Methods included lecture, demonstrations, audience participation activities, group discussion, and individual consultation on diet problems. Follow-up evaluation two weeks after the workshop showed that 70% of the respondents had altered their dietary patterns and/or experienced weight loss as a result of changes made following the program.

Although nutrition specialist models for delivering nutrition education to older populations have been the most prevalent, peer education models have recently emerged as a viable option. Shannon, Smiciklas-

Wright, Davis, and Lewis (1983) report the development of a program that recruited and trained 22 older adults to create interest in nutrition among their peers and to serve as liaisons between peers and sound sources of nutrition information and expertise. The program, which was conducted in Pennsylvania with assistance from Cooperative Extension, reached a total of 933 participants. Although no impact data regarding change in dietary habits were reported, the evaluations showed that sessions were well organized and interesting and provided information useful to the participants' daily lives. In addition, the majority of the volunteers said that the experience was a good one and that the peer education approach should be continued in nutrition education for the elderly.

A similar program on a larger scale was conducted by Cohen (1992); 90 older adult volunteers were recruited and trained by Massachusetts Cooperative Extension personnel. More than 2,500 seniors participated in peer-led workshops, and an additional 1,950 were reached through health fairs staffed by volunteers. Impact data showed substantial increase in nutrition knowledge (81% correct scores on the posttest, compared with 68% correct on the pretest), and the majority of participants improved their diets and food practices (64% reduced sodium, 69% increased fiber, and 79% improved food safety practices). Volunteers grew in their self-esteem as a result of the project, and many chose to volunteer for longer than the original time commitment requested.

Lee, Grant, and Gillis's (1987) peer education project focused on educating seniors in nutrition, consumer issues, and proper use of medication, using 167 older adult volunteers. Using a one-group, pretest/posttest evaluation design, the researchers found that there was an increase in participants' knowledge in all content areas, a decrease in participants' beliefs in nutrition myths, and a decrease in self-perceived loneliness. As with the two previous programs, the senior volunteers reported personal gains from their involvement in the program.

Although successfully implemented, both nutrition specialist and peer education models for delivering nutrition education to the elderly appear to have some limitations. For example, the nutrition education programs using lesson formats ranging from multiweek programs to one-day efforts show that, for the most part, the nutrition specialist model has had little success in changing diet behaviors. Most of the studies reviewed show the most change in cognitive behavior, with less success in actual changing of food choice and food consumption behaviors. Some of the studies demonstrate the difficulties in trying to do the latter, particularly from a methodological standpoint. Food recalls and other subjective means of determining food consumption have obvious drawbacks. Moreover, considering that some of the studies on urban populations incorporated quasi-experimental design, one can imagine the problems that might be encountered in attempting to use these designs in isolated rural areas, where logistical challenges are the norm.

The peer education models may have more promise. Clearly, more older adults can be reached when a large cadre of volunteers is trained and can work with groups of seniors. This model may be particularly effective in rural areas, where volunteers could go to senior centers and clubs in small towns and also organize meetings in people's homes. Impact data show that, as with the nutrition specialist model, the peer model increases nutrition knowledge and, in one case, changed dietary behavior. However, stronger evaluation designs must be incorporated in peer education programs to determine if delivery of nutrition education by peers can really make a difference in older adults' diet and food practices.

Service Delivery Models

Service delivery models that provide food services to elders include group feeding programs such as those sponsored by Title III-C of the Older Americans Act, home-delivered meals, homemaker services, and food stamps. Although the literature on the effectiveness of these programs is more abundant than is the case for nutrition education programs, there has still been little research conducted on rural populations. Thus the effectiveness of food programs for general older populations will be discussed, with attention given to those studies on rural elderly where available.

Congregate meal programs funded through Title III-C1 of the Older Americans Act are actually more available in rural areas than in urban areas, although urban programs serve more meals (Kirschner Associates, 1981). In spring 1980 there were 1,155 nutrition projects administering food service at nearly 12,000 congregate meal sites. The majority of the nutrition projects (64%) and meal sites (57%) were in rural settings. Although there were more rural projects, the urban projects served many more meals, approximately twice as many per day as served by rural projects. In addition to their availability, differences have been found in the quality of meals and sanitation of nutrition sites in rural areas compared with urban areas (Kirschner Associates, 1981).

Problems still prevail, however, in rural congregate meal programs because of lack of adequate transportation, inability to reach isolated rural elderly in remote areas, and high costs of operation of sites (Farmers Home Administration, 1980). Nevertheless, in studies of both rural and urban elderly, those who use congregate meal programs have generally had better diets than those who do not.

Kirschner Associates (1981) have conducted the most extensive evaluations of the Elderly Nutrition Program (ENP). In 1976, four years after the inception of ENP, the Administration on Aging commissioned a national study of the program. The second phase of the study focused on the extent to which services significantly benefited older Americans. With a study design that included visits to 70 meal sites and a survey of 250 staff and 2,000 participants, the researchers found that the program was meeting a principal goal of enhancing nutrient intake, and that increased nutrient intake, particularly of calcium, was directly related to program participation.

Other studies support the findings by Kirschner Associates regarding the effectiveness of congregate meals. Kohrs (1978) compared the diets of 154 elders in central Missouri who had eaten at a meal site on a given day with those of 200 who had not. The findings showed that those who ate the program meal consumed a significantly higher percentage of the recommended dietary allowances for energy, protein, and calcium than did those who did not consume the program meal. Holahan and Kunkel (1986) studied 69 nutrition site participants in South Carolina to determine the contribution of the congregate meal to their nutrient intake. The findings showed that overall nutrient intake was adequate (i.e., mean intakes of all nutrients exceeding 67% of RDA), and lunches supplied 33% of total nutrient intake whether they were program meals or lunches at home. However, the researchers found that, for some participants, the program lunch supplied up to 90% of the total intake, underscoring the importance of the congregate meal for some elderly.

Other studies suggest that the congregate meal may be less effective in affecting the overall diets of the elderly. Posner (1979), who analyzed the influence of congregate meals on a sample of older adults in the Boston area, found that less than 5% reported that the program had an impact on their health or diet. Balsam and Rogers (1991) report an earlier study in Massachusetts by Balsam and others that compared 65 program participants with 60 matched controls who did not participate in the meal program. No significant differences were found between participants and nonparticipants in their intake of foods from the four food groups.

Studies are less available regarding the effectiveness of other food-related services, and their results are mixed. Guthrie et al. (1972) found that low-income rural elderly food stamp recipients in Pennsylvania, in comparison with nonrecipients, had improved intakes of energy, protein, and iron. In contrast, as a part of a study to investigate impacts of cash payments for food coupons among elderly recipients, Posner, Ohls, and Morgan (1987) studied a sample of program recipients ($n = 1,400$) and eligible nonrecipients ($n = 500$) from six sites and found that food stamps did not produce statistically significant improvements in nutrient intake. With regard to home-delivered meals, Steele and Bryan (1985-1986) found that homebound elderly nonrecipients generally seemed to fare better in nutrient intake than did recipients of the service. These authors conclude that the provision of nutrition services to homebound elderly appears to be lagging behind need, and encourage further study of this problem.

There appear to be a couple of important trends in the findings regarding the effectiveness of food-related services for older populations. First, of the food-related services reviewed, congregate meals are the most effective for improving the diets and food practices of seniors, as indicated by the studies conducted by Kirschner Associates (1981), Kohrs (1978), and Holahan and Kunkel (1986). Second, in those studies of effectiveness of food-related services where positive outcomes on diet and food practices were reported, all were conducted in rural areas (e.g., congregate meal studies in Missouri and South Carolina and a food stamp study in Pennsylvania). This may suggest that food-related services are more successful in changing the food behaviors of elderly in rural areas than in urban areas, although clearly additional research would need to be conducted to support this tentative conclusion. Nevertheless, the fact that food-related services do appear to have a positive impact on rural elderly is encouraging and speaks well of program delivery in rural areas.

There are, however, instances where practitioners involved in nutrition programs discover barriers in delivering services to rural elderly. These barriers are evident in both food-related service programs and nutrition education programs. One of the major barriers to delivering nutrition programs to rural elderly, and in fact to any elderly audience, is that changing the eating habits of older adults can be difficult, because food behavior patterns have been determined over a period of years. As a result, rural elders may be less likely to consume certain foods and may not be receptive to other nutrition programming—or at least not to the point of changing behavior. In dealing with this issue, practitioners may have some discomfort in attempting to deliver nutrition programs—for example, they may feel it is a little presumptuous to give dietary guidelines to octogenarians. In these instances, it is important to help learners to expand their food awareness and modify existing habits, but with respect for their lifelong food preferences.

Because of their age as well as other reasons, rural elderly participants of nutrition programs may lack motivation for learning about nutrition, another barrier to program delivery. Reduction in energy, vision and hearing impairment, and chronic illnesses can make older adults less receptive to educational endeavors (Peterson, 1983). Thus implementing programs in an interesting, receptive format can be a challenge. There is considerable evidence that interactive formats such as minidemonstrations, television, and even computers can be used effectively with older audiences (Ralston, 1986a). Major principles to consider in effective nutrition education delivery with older learners include challenging and stimulating participants rather than patronizing them, keeping programs short and concise in length and humorous and entertaining in delivery, and providing ways for learners to use various sensory modes to learn (seeing, hearing, tasting, touching, smelling) (Peterson, 1983).

Providing Nutrition Services: Problems and Needed Programs

We have pointed out several challenges inherent in delivering nutrition services to rural elderly, including (a) the existence of certain populations at greatest risk, such as those who are older, male, and black and who have lower incomes; (b) rural values that embrace traditional ideas about food preparation and quality and endorse independence and "making do," even to the extent of cutting food purchases to accommodate income limitations; (c) problems in getting access to food, such as transportation to obtain food as well as health problems and physical conditions that may hamper mobility; and (d) the low number of services in general, although there has been an increase in some food-related services such as congregate meals and homemakers.

Although these challenges are prevalent in delivering nutrition services to rural elderly, there are indications of program successes. Clearly, food-related services, particularly congregate meals, have been found to have positive impacts on rural elders' diets and food practices. Nutrition education for rural elderly appears to have more potential for affecting dietary behavior when peers are used in program delivery than when nutrition specialists are used. Age, lack of interest in nutrition, resistance to changing dietary behavior, and physical decline that may affect learning are barriers that must be taken into consideration in delivering nutritional services to rural elderly populations. Addressing these challenges and barriers and building on program successes will not be easy, particularly considering the decreased local funding in both rural and urban areas for human services, and the increased attention to urban problems in general.

In seeking solutions, we must assume that, for the near future, there will be scarce resources both locally and nationally; as a result, few new programs will be developed to serve elderly populations, particularly rural elderly. With limited resources, it will be important to use existing programs and find ways to be creative in using these programs to meet the needs of rural clientele. Moreover, consideration should be given to building on the strengths of rural elderly. In fact, in these increasingly difficult times, when government support is dwindling, rural elderly's independence and reliance on natural helping networks (family and friends) in times of need are two important strengths on which to build.

The independence of rural elders and their sometime resistance to new programs can be useful if practitioners study, in a more in-depth way, the existing services that rural people themselves have already created. Coward (1979) points out that certain organizations have been able to establish credibility in providing family-oriented services and thus have been accepted by rural residents. The existing nutrition network in rural areas includes not only food-related services such as congregate meals, home-delivered meals, homemaker service, and food stamps, but also established rural organizations—churches, public schools, Cooperative Extension, and social clubs, among others. Stronger linkages need to be developed within the nutrition network that would bring greater recognition of the nutrition needs of rural elders, expand the populations that might be reached, and address the problem of limited professional staff in rural areas (Coward, 1979). For example, use of volunteers for delivering nutrition education to the elderly, perhaps organized by Cooperative Extension, could include not only peers but also high school students enrolled in nutrition classes, church members, and extension volunteers. These groups might work with both government-sponsored food programs and senior clubs and other grassroots senior organizations, which often have competing senior programming in small rural communities (Ralston, 1986b). Community organizations that collectively take on service projects as "organizational volunteers" can be very effective in providing outreach to frail rural elderly (Young, Goughler, & Larson, 1986).

Natural helpers, such as family, friends, and neighbors, who are used by rural elderly in times of need, are another strength of this group and are clearly key individuals who should be informed about both nutrition education and the service delivery system. Coward (1979) points out that, many times, human service program planners fail to recognize that the recipients of their services are embedded in a social context. He argues that a family-oriented approach should be used that includes involving the helper in increasing the impact of the service (i.e., encouraging use of the service) and in serving as a support to the professional staff. One means of informing natural helpers in rural areas about nutrition education and the service delivery system is through educational efforts that bring those with expertise to rural communities. One-day workshops, which have been successfully implemented in rural areas, might be one means of bringing in-depth information to natural helpers on a short-term basis (Hausafus, Ralston, & DeLanoit, 1985; Ralston & Jones, 1984).

Natural helpers can also be more broadly defined as gatekeepers or nontraditional referral sources trained to identify and locate high-risk elderly who would not self-refer and who do not have relatives or others to act on their behalf (Raschko, 1985). Gatekeepers include, for example, rural mail carriers, veterinarians, extension service workers, grocers, pharmacists, and friends. The use of gatekeepers appears to be a particularly effective way of enhancing service delivery to older people in rural areas, because elderly persons, particularly those in isolated areas, may not only find out about a service but also may be convinced to use the service because someone they trust has recommended it (Atkinson & Stuck, 1991; Buckwalter, Smith, Zevenbergen, & Russell, 1991).

This discussion has clearly emphasized using existing programs in creative ways to meet the nutritional needs of rural elderly. Few new resources will be available for social programs, thus the allocation of present resources will be of priority in the 1990s. This translates into strengthening political efforts to increase the awareness of the critical needs in rural areas as our society is faced with a wealth of social and economic ills in urban areas. Thus providing nutritional services to rural elderly will increasingly become a political effort, and that is the focus of the final section of this chapter.

Policy Issues and Research Needs

Nutrition policy issues for the rural elderly must be discussed within the context of rural America in the past two decades. Flora and Christenson (1991) point out that, whereas the 1970s brought a rural renaissance, the 1980s were a decade of rural decline and turnback. In the 1980s rural areas, in comparison with urban areas, were characterized by economic decline, including higher unemployment, lower job growth rates, decreased family income, increased out-migration, and greater increase in poverty. Macroeconomic developments such as tight monetary policy, reduced taxes, and deregulation contributed to this economic decline. As the rural environment slipped into further decay, few social policies were developed to solve problems created by the economic decline. Women, the poor, the aged, and minorities in rural areas were often those disenfranchised by economic decline and the lack of social policy development. Flora and Christenson (1991) conclude that the 1990s will be a decade of decision for U.S. leaders: "Either we will have two Americas, geographically and economically distinct, with the rural one considerably disadvantaged compared to the urban one, or efforts will be made to promote equity and opportunities for rural people in rural areas" (p. 1).

Within this context of rural America in recent years, policy issues regarding the elderly have been almost nonexistent. As Kaiser (1991) points out, "In the 1980s, rural aging issues were 'left off the list' of the federal agenda" (p. 133). A rural aging agenda, however, is beginning to reappear, with some of the rekindled interest in areas related to health. Some examples include the establishment of the Office of Rural Health Policy in the U.S. Department of Health and Human Services and, for a brief period, the funding of the National Resource Center on Rural Elderly by the Administration on Aging.

Other examples demonstrate the broad concern for health promotion among the elderly as well as the general public. The Office of Disease Prevention and Health Promotion in the Department of Health and

Human Services has coordinated publication of materials to promote good health among all Americans, including the elderly (e.g., *Surgeon General's Report on Nutrition and Health, Healthy People 2000,* and *Dietary Guidelines for Americans*) (J. M. McGinnis, personal communication, 1992). The National Cancer Institute, in conjunction with the produce industry, launched its "5 a Day—for Better Health" program in 1992 to promote consumption of five to nine servings of fruits and vegetables each day (Community Nutrition Institute, 1992). Finally, the Health Promotion Institute (HPI) of the National Council on the Aging (NCOA) was founded in 1990 to provide a forum for professionals who are involved in senior wellness education, programming, and research (Center on Rural Elderly, 1991a). NCOA/HPI has advocated the inclusion of health promotion and preventive services in the Older Americans Act, and has collaborated with other organizations on a five-year campaign to promote nutrition assessment and intervention for older people in the health care and social services systems (Center on Rural Elderly, 1991a).

These examples, although not all-inclusive, are encouraging in that there appears to be major awareness of health and nutrition needs, not only of the elderly, but of the general public as well. A concern that lingers, however, is the extent to which these efforts are reaching rural elderly, particularly those most at risk. Balsam and Rogers (1991) speak to this issue in their discussion of how the Elderly Nutrition Program has failed to reach the "socially impaired"—the disabled, those without transportation, the poorest of the poor, the very old, and members of certain minority groups. Although they do not specifically mention the rural elderly, the populations outlined are often those found in rural areas.

Flora and Christenson (1991) argue that policies for rural America need to be targeted policies, based on the problem a policy is designed to address. A particular issue in aging circles is whether or not the Older Americans Act should be refocused to serve those older people with the greatest social and economic need rather than all older people who meet a certain age criterion (Center on Rural Elderly, 1991b; Skinner, 1990; Stanford, 1990). Data would support targeting populations, considering the lack of use of services by at-risk elderly and the decline in the elderly poverty rate (Community Nutrition Institute, 1992). As Kaiser (1991) points out, rural elderly could benefit from targeting policies if provisions were made in the Older Americans Act "to recognize the paucity of providers, ensure fair distribution of resources for rural areas, and support the added costs of delivering services in low-density, high distance areas" (pp. 136-137). Clearly, the fate of rural elderly and rural people in general will be determined by the degree to which our society recognizes the inequities in policies between rural and urban America.

Research can be one means of strengthening policy development for rural elderly. This chapter has pointed out some salient research needs in both problems to be investigated and methodology. First, it is clear that research is needed on nutritional status of rural elderly, with attention to determining those subgroups that might be at high risk for poor nutritional status. Many of the studies conducted thus far on nutritional status of the elderly have included only small, local samples. Broader-based studies with larger populations would allow for investigation of nutritional status of subgroups, more powerful statistical analyses, and greater generalizability. The National Health and Nutrition Examination Survey (NHANES II), conducted from 1976 to 1980, studied the overall health status of the U.S. population from age 6 to 74, including 8,080 who were 55 to 74 years of age. This study is limited, however, because of the exclusion of those over 74 years of age. With NHANES III under way, which will include those over 74 years of age, there will be opportunities for researchers to conduct broader-based studies and to make rural/urban as well as other comparisons.

Another area of research that needs to be strengthened involves the determination of the effectiveness of nutrition education with rural elderly populations. Few of the studies concerning the effectiveness of nutrition education described in this chapter included rural elderly samples. In addition, few studies used rigorous designs that incorporated measures determining behavior change in food consumption and practices of this population. Because many innovative nutrition education programs are initiated by practitioners, care will need to be taken to include research expertise on a collaborative basis in this programming. Such efforts would not only strengthen the evaluations of these programs but would also assist researchers by broadening their perspectives on how nutrition education can be implemented.

Summary and Conclusions

This chapter has addressed nutrition and the rural elderly, demonstrating that there is indeed a need for nutritional services for this group. Although the evidence regarding nutritional status of rural elderly is sparse, data that are available show that certain subgroups are at greater nutritional risk—those who are older, male, and black and who have lower incomes. Factors related to nutrition and rural elderly include (a) traditional values about food and conservative financial practices, which can affect the amount of money allocated toward food; (b) access to food, which is characterized by availability of formal food-related services but complicated by transportation and other logistical problems; and (c) dependence of the elderly on family, friends, and neighbors for food acquisition and preparation when needed.

Strategies for intervention for providing nutritional services to rural elderly include nutrition education by nutrition specialists and peers and service programs provided through congregate meals, homemaker services, and food stamps and other government-sponsored programs. Peer nutrition education programs may be an effective way of reaching rural elderly because of the possibility of including diverse groups of outreach workers and volunteers. Stronger impact data, however, need to be collected before we can determine the degree to which these programs can change nutritional behavior in rural elderly populations. Congregate meal programs consistently appear to be the most effective food service in improving diets and food practices of seniors. Future programs for delivering nutritional services need to build on the strengths of rural elderly, including their independence and reliance on natural helpers. Moreover, with limited resources locally and nationally, broadened nutrition networks that include collaboration between natural helpers and formal services need to be developed to meet nutritional needs of this group. Of major importance, however, is the development of policies that generally would rectify the inequities between rural and urban America and more specifically would target elderly populations with the greatest social and economic need. Clearly, current evidence suggests that the rural elderly, with at-risk subgroups and an environment that has recently suffered from further social and economic decline, should be one of these targeted populations.

11

Home Health Services
in Rural America

LINDA J. REDFORD
ALISON B. SEVERNS

The need to reexamine and rethink how health and supportive services are organized and delivered in the United States takes on particular urgency when one considers our aging population. The costs of long-term care are impoverishing many elderly and their families. Although older people prefer to live out their lives in their own homes, they often find it impossible to identify, obtain, and afford the home care services they need to stay in their homes.

Home care includes a variety of services, some of which focus on the health or medical needs of older persons and others of which are designed to provide assistance with the routine daily activities necessary to independent living. The health, or "medical," model of services includes skilled nursing care, home health aide care, and therapies for recuperative and rehabilitative care. Supportive services, or "social" model services, can include homemaker services, chore services, meal services, personal care, respite care, and a variety of other services oriented around daily tasks. If provided in a timely and appropriate fashion, home care services can alleviate or delay the need for institutional care among older persons experiencing acute or chronic functional impairments.

Need for Services in the Home

In few areas of this country is the need for in-home health and supportive services greater than in rural America. Small towns have a higher proportion of elderly than do urban areas, 13% versus 11%, and in towns of 2,500 to 10,000 this proportion is often 15% or greater (U.S. Bureau of the Census, 1983b). In some rural counties, the proportion of elderly is greater than 25%. More important, a large and growing number of these elderly are 85 years of age and older (U.S. Bureau of the Census, 1981). At such advanced ages, people have much greater vulnerability to chronic illness and disability. This suggests that access to community-based and in-home long-term care services is now, and will continue to be, an important issue for rural communities.

Studies of the health and functional status of rural elderly support this contention. Rural elderly tend to have more chronic health impairments (Office of Technology Assessment, 1990), higher numbers of medical conditions, more functional limitations, and a greater number of performance difficulties in activities of daily living and instrumental activities of daily living than do urban elderly (Coward, 1991; Coward & Dwyer, 1991b; Ecosometrics, 1981). However, when factors such as age, sex, income, living arrangement, and education are controlled, many of these differences disappear (Cutler & Coward, 1988; Krout, 1991b). These findings suggest that differences in health status between urban and rural elderly may reflect sociocultural characteristics of the persons residing in rural areas, rather than the environment per se (Coward & Cutler, 1988). For example, we know that rural elderly are more likely than urban elderly to be poor, to have substandard housing, and to have fewer options in formal services (Coward & Lee, 1985a). All of these are factors that tend to be associated with poorer health status.

Differences in health status are not, however, uniformly related to urban or rural residence (Cooper, 1988; Coward & Cutler, 1989; Cutler & Coward, 1988). The greatest extremes in health status have been found in nonmetropolitan areas. "Farm" dwellers have been found to be among the healthiest of any elderly population group, whereas the elderly in small rural towns experience the most numerous and most debilitating health problems (Coward & Cutler, 1988). The reasons for these differences are not clear. It may be a difference in the sociocultural characteristics of persons residing in small towns, a reflection of migratory patterns of persons experiencing health and functional impairments, or the result of less obvious factors. Certainly, it is a finding deserving of further study.

Service Access and Availability

Service availability is defined as the presence of a service within a specific geographic area or defined population. In the 1970s and early 1980s, a number of studies reported marked differences between urban and rural communities in availability of health and social services, with rural communities having narrower ranges and fewer alternatives for in-home services (Coward & Cutler, 1989; Krout, 1986; Nelson, 1980). However, as early as the mid-1970s, there were indications that service availability was improving in rural communities (Taietz & Milton, 1979). This gap is likely to have narrowed even more in the past decade, with the implementation of Medicaid waivers and the expansion of home care services under Title III of the Older Americans Act.

Recent studies provide some support for this contention. In a study of 105 Kansas counties, Gibbons, Camp, and Kaiser (1991) found some rural counties with relatively complete long-term care service continua. Although there was considerable variation among rural areas, some nonmetropolitan counties had a wider range of long-term care services than can be found in some metropolitan communities.

Kenney and Dubay (1992) found that rural areas have more home health agencies per population than do urban areas. Although another study showed these rural agencies to have about half the staff numbers of urban agencies, 11.5 compared with 23.7, they still had a slightly higher ratio of full-time staff members to every 100 elders than did urban agencies, 2.9 versus 2.6 (Hoyer, 1988).

The issue of access extends beyond the existence of a particular service to actual usage patterns relating to the service. Factors that influence access to services are numerous; they include geographic distance and topography, financial ability to purchase services, knowledge of services, eligibility constraints, and willingness to utilize existing services.

In spite of there being more home health agencies per population in rural than urban areas, there is evidence of lesser access to home health services among rural elderly. Even when numerous potential intervening factors were considered, Kenney and Dubay (1992) found that Medicare beneficiaries in rural areas were 17% less likely to use home health benefits than were those in urban areas. It is unclear whether this difference is the result of differences in availability of *needed* services, differences in attitudinal and behavioral characteristics of urban and rural elderly, differences in referral patterns, or other factors not yet identified.

Rural elderly are also less likely to get physical therapy, occupational therapy, and some of the other therapies offered under the Medicare program (Institute of Medicine, 1989). It is unclear whether this is the result of a lack of therapists in rural communities, a difference in the needs of rural home health patients, or the fact that there are too few persons needing therapy to make it feasible for rural agencies to employ or contract with therapists. Another possibility is that some therapies, at least those that are relatively routine, may be provided by other health workers, such as home health nurses.

Usage patterns relating to social model services are much more difficult to obtain. Reporting requirements relating to federal and state monies used for the more socially oriented services are inadequate or nonexistent. Even less information is available on services and the persons served in programs funded through Social Services Block Grants and other state administered programs.

Rural Home Care: Standard and Alternative Approaches

Traditional Approaches

Financing is a major driving and shaping force in our current formal service system. The types of services provided, the persons authorized to provide the services, and the ways in which services are delivered are largely dictated and enforced through the structure and regulations of reimbursement sources. Government funding for in-home services for the elderly comes primarily from Medicare, Medicaid, Social Services Block Grants, and the Older Americans Act. State monies are increasingly being targeted for community-based and in-home services in attempts to contain the escalating costs of institutional care, but state monies still make up a small percentage of home care dollars.

The types of care covered, eligibility for services, and the duration of services vary among these payment sources. Although the range of services offered under Medicare, Medicaid, Title XX, Title III, Veterans Administration, and state funds may seem impressive, in reality it is not. Medicare covers 37% of publicly financed in-home care costs, but this represents less than 4% of total Medicare expenditures. Medicaid covers 47% of publicly financed home care, and other federal and state programs together cover 16% (Pepper Commission, 1990). Regardless of the source, the percentage of actual costs of in-home care covered through public monies is minuscule. Home care, particularly long-term care, is largely provided by family and friends or financed out of pocket by the elderly or their families.

Medicare. Medicare is a major source of funding for skilled nursing care and therapies in the home. Persons served under Medicare monies must meet several criteria, including being confined to the home (homebound). The services covered under Medicare include part-time or intermittent skilled nursing, physical therapy, and speech therapy. If one or more of these services are needed, Medicare will also cover occupational therapy, home health aide services, medical social services, medical supplies, and durable medical equipment. Support services, such as laundry, meal preparation, shopping, and other domestic and home maintenance, are not covered.

To be reimbursed by Medicare, the agency providing the services must be participating in Medicare and must meet Medicare provider certification requirements. Some rural home health agencies and local health departments have had difficulty complying with Medicare regulations because they lack a full-time registered nurse director or have difficulty affording and justifying a full-time RN solely for home health services (Office of Technology Assessment, 1990).

Medicaid. Medicaid is a federally aided program in which state matching monies are required and the state assumes program administration responsibilities. Aged are "categorically eligible" for Medicaid if their income levels are low enough to meet the state's eligibility criteria. The federal government sets some minimum standards for eligibility and services, but states vary greatly in Medicaid eligibility requirements, services offered, and payment levels and procedures for providers.

The majority of Medicaid funds spent on elderly individuals are spent for nursing home care. However, the Title XIX Home and Community-Based Waiver Program allows states to use Medicaid monies for in-home services for those individuals who are Medicaid eligible and require nursing home-level care. A wide range of services can be provided under these programs, but these services are available only to the most indigent and disabled sector of the elderly population, and the expenditures for services cannot exceed the cost of Medicaid reimbursement to nursing homes.

Title XX of the Social Security Act. Title XX authorizes reimbursement to states for social services provided through Social Services Block Grants. States have the flexibility to spend these monies based on needs as identified by the state, including such services as adult day care, protective services, counseling, respite care, homemaker services, home-delivered and congregate meals, transportation, and many others.

The eligibility criteria for these services vary from state to state, as do determinations regarding copayments and user fees. Generally, these services are targeted to lower-income individuals. As federal reporting is no longer required, it is very difficult to ascertain how, to whom, and for what these monies are allocated within states.

Title III of the Older Americans Act. Title III of the Older Americans Act provides monies for supportive services and senior centers, congregate and home-delivered meals, and case management. Under supportive services, Area Agencies on Aging can fund such services as transportation, homemaker services, personal care, chore services, health services, respite care, case management, and a variety of other services needed for independent living. All persons 60 years of age and older are eligible for these services, regardless of income. Nevertheless, special emphasis is supposed to be placed on targeting low-income, minority, and isolated older people.

Veterans Administration funds. The VA system provides a variety of community-based and in-home services. Some of these services are based out of VA medical centers in towns serving rural areas, but are available only to veterans who qualify for services. Services available in the VA system include hospital-based home care teams, respite care, and adult day health care.

State funds. Faced with a growing demand for long-term care services, rising institutional costs, and the reluctance of the federal government to make any significant commitment to community-based and in-home services, states have been forced to fund noninstitutional long-term care services through state general revenues and monies from special taxation, lotteries, and other revenue-producing mechanisms. The services funded include in-home supportive services, such as homemaker, personal care, and chore services. Occasionally, community-based services, such as adult day care and senior centers, also receive state and local monies. In most cases, some form of case management function is financed under state programs to ensure appropriate and cost-effective use of services.

Alternative Models

Social/health maintenance organizations. In recent years, the Health Care Financing Administration has provided waivers for demonstration projects to allow Medicare, Medicaid, and other federal monies to be used for some in-home long-term care services (Hughes, 1986; Leutz et al., 1985). As an extension of the health maintenance organization (HMO) concept, the social/health maintenance organizations (S/HMOs) were developed. S/HMOs are intended to provide a complete range of social and health maintenance services under a fixed capitation fee through a nonprofit provider organization. Acute hospital care, nursing home care, ambulatory medical care, and personal care support services, including home health, homemaker, and chore services, are provided by or through the S/HMO for a fixed annual prepaid capitation fee.

This approach has not been applied strictly to rural areas. As with HMOs, which draw enrollees from larger population bases in rural communities, the S/HMO model faces problems with attaining an adequate and diversified enrollment base. Even if regional approaches are used, factors of poverty, poor health, distance, and the reluctance of rural populations to become involved with "untried" models might pose obstacles. Still, it is a model that provides the possibility of better access to home care than current financing mechanisms.

On-Lok model. On-Lok, a community-based program in San Francisco, embarked on an experiment several years ago to provide risk-based prepaid long-term care to an exclusively high-risk elderly population. All enrollees in the program are eligible for skilled nursing facility (SNF) care. For the first 100 days of enrollment, Medicare pays On-Lok the SNF rate for care. After 100 days, On-Lok receives the Medicaid rate or the client pays approximately $1,000 per month for care until the Medicaid spend-down level is met. There is a heavy emphasis on adult day care, but the benefits are quite comprehensive, including hospital care, nursing home care, medical and specialty care, and home care.

At present, there are several communities serving as sites for replications of the On-Lok model, but few of the sites serve rural populations. The South Carolina site, which serves some rural elderly, has found that, with the primary emphasis on adult day care, transportation poses a problem for rural residents. If rural hospitals and other providers diversify their services to offer adult day care in rural communities, this might alleviate some of the transportation problems and increase the likelihood of this being a viable model for rural communities.

State and local models. States and local communities have been the innovators in instituting long-term care reform, through both creative financing and reorganization of home care services. Numerous states now provide in-home care for elderly through state and/or local revenues or through a combination of local, state, and federal monies, usually Medicaid, Title XX, and/or Title III. Most states have continued to rely on Medicare and Medicaid for home health services while using state monies to increase the types and amounts of supportive services, particularly homemaker, personal care, and chore services.

Wisconsin and Oregon are examples of states that have implemented quite comprehensive long-term care programs. Both states have consolidated all components of their long-term care programs into a single administrative structure at the state level and a highly integrated delivery system at the local level. In Wisconsin, the core of the program is state monies, whereas the Oregon program has been built largely around federal monies, the Medicaid Home and Community-Based Waiver Program (Justice & Preston, 1986).

The Wisconsin program, called the Community Options Program (COP), has more flexibility because of the state money core. It is the focal point for the coordination of all federal, state, and local resources devoted to community care services and serves all disabled, including the mentally ill and chemically dependent. There are no mandated or disallowed services. There is a strong emphasis on client involvement and choice in all aspects of the program. The Oregon program, on the other hand, is focused solely on the elderly and the services provided must be in accordance with federal guidelines.

Administrative control of Wisconsin's COP is at the county level. Each county is required to have a local planning committee, including at least five consumers of services, to develop a county COP plan. This approach is consistent with a long history of state-supervised and county-administered human services delivery in Wisconsin. In contrast,

Oregon's human service system has historically been under strong state control. With the introduction of the waiver, the system changed to one of state supervision with local program management. This was not done without significant tension and disagreement among various levels of government, service providers, and aging advocacy groups. Through a process of meetings and consensus building, however, the problems were overcome.

The Oregon program is particularly noteworthy because of the conditions under which it developed. The entire state system was reorganized and a Medicaid Home and Community-Based Waiver put in place in a relatively short time and in a period of serious financial constraints. A severe economic recession began to affect Oregon at about the time the state's long-term care initiative was implemented. This meant tight cost controls and considerable pressure on community service systems. The system has survived and become a model, in large part because leaders in the state were willing to "take risks and persevere" (Justice & Preston, 1986).

Community Approaches to Developing and Integrating Health and Social Services

Centralization and Diversification of Services

One approach communities have used to simplify and expand their health and social care systems is to integrate services under one administrative structure or, at least, in a central location. The following are some examples of centralization and diversification.

Rural hospitals. Rural hospitals have closed in record numbers over the past 10 years as a result of low occupancy rates and shrinking markets. Many rural hospitals are in or heading for serious financial difficulties and must change their missions and service structures or close (Office of Technology Assessment, 1990). Faced with the possible closure of a community hospital and the loss of what is often a major employer, communities have begun to work more closely with the hospitals to find ways to maintain them in a form that better serves the needs of the community. Because reimbursement potential is a critical factor in the selection of services, home health care has been a logical choice. In 1988, hospital-based Medicare-certified home health agencies accounted for 32% of all rural versus 25% of all urban home health agencies.

Rural hospitals also have potential as focal points for the provision of a more integrated service delivery system. As these facilities reduce acute hospital beds, they can serve as sites for either housing in-home provider organizations or actually becoming the administrative provider of these services, particularly the services that do not already exist or are too limited to meet the demand. By locating services in one place or providing an administrative umbrella over health and supportive services, these hospitals may accomplish better integration and coordination of services. Although colocation of providers does not guarantee better coordination, it does tend to reduce some of the physical barriers to communication and cooperation among providers.

Rural nursing homes. Rural nursing homes may also be logical sites for colocating home health and supportive service providers or may serve as developers and providers of such services. Although there are few models for this in the United States, some Canadian nursing homes have been providers of in-home services for many years. Of course, it must also be recognized that the Canadian health care system reimburses a wide variety of in-home health and supportive services.

Community health centers. Community health centers (CHCs) have been one of the federally supported mainstays of rural health in human resource shortage areas. Begun under the 1975 Rural Health Initiative as part of the federally supported Community Health Centers Program, there are now 488 such centers in rural areas across the country (Smith & Zuckerman, 1991). These centers are required to provide basic primary care services, such as physician services, laboratory and radiology, preventive health services, emergency medical services, and transportation. In addition, CHCs may provide home health services and long-term care services, when appropriate.

As with rural hospitals and other rural providers, CHCs are facing financial and other pressures. CHCs are heavily dependent on government grant funding to cover expenses and are looking at diversification as one way to maintain financial viability. By the mid-1980s, many CHCs had started expanding into optional services or initiating coordination with other community organizations (Wood, Hughes, & Estes, 1986). The elderly are a particularly attractive target group for CHCs because of Medicare reimbursement for many home health services.

The degree to which CHCs will move into supportive services, which are less likely to be reimbursed, remains to be seen.

Coordination of Existing Services

Case management has emerged as a mechanism for guiding the use of limited public and private resources to care for functionally impaired older persons. Case management is a process that includes, in its most basic form, an assessment of needs, development of a service plan, and the implementation and monitoring of that plan on behalf of a client. In some places the case manager is responsible for eligibility determination and service authorization. Professional case managers have also been shown to be effective in the role of resource developers, bringing together informal and formal resources in ways that maximize the effectiveness of both.

Professional Human Resources

Rural communities face a scarcity of professional providers and a need for professionals who can perform effectively with a much higher level of autonomy and flexibility than is required in most urban areas. The providers available in rural communities often lack the educational background to perform most effectively in rural home care. For example, many of the nurses in rural communities have been educated in programs that provide little or no community health experience. Yet, community health nursing skills, with a strong focus on primary care, case management, and long-term care, are vital in rural communities. On the other hand, in our university health provider programs, specialization has overshadowed the more generalist focus needed to function in rural communities. Therapists, social workers, and other in-home providers must also be aware of and prepared to deal with the nuances of rural practice, and few educational programs prepare them for this area.

A number of strategies are now being employed that will better prepare those currently practicing in rural communities and will increase the numbers of well-prepared professional service providers. Collaborative linkages among community colleges, universities, and other educational institutions are providing resources for training, continuing education, and consultive support needed by health and social services professionals, ancillary support personnel, and voluntary caregivers.

Cooperation among educational providers of all levels is also particularly important to advancing educational opportunities in rural communities. The linkages developed among educational institutions should provide logical and attainable career ladders for all levels of community providers. Demands from communities and the willingness of communities to support the education and employment of community residents in areas of need may be the impetus needed to get career ladder approaches out of the quagmire in which many have languished for the past two decades.

There are several educational models for advancing the knowledge of rural providers. Many colleges and universities provide continuing education programs for professionals and ancillary personnel in rural communities. Area health education centers in several rural states, in collaboration with major state universities, provide continuing education and opportunities for closer collaboration between urban and rural health providers.

Under funding from the Bureau of Health Professions of the U.S. Department of Health and Human Services, a number of universities have established geriatric education centers and now provide geriatric and gerontological education for urban and rural health providers at state and regional levels. In addition to providing educational offerings in rural communities, rural providers also have the opportunity to spend extended amounts of time in university hospitals, clinics, and community settings to update their knowledge in care of the elderly.

It has been clearly shown that recruitment and retention of professional health personnel in rural areas is best accomplished by educating persons already living in those areas. Recruiting and even paying the tuition for bright and motivated ancillary workers from the community to continue their education in nursing, social services, allied health fields, or other needed professions is more likely to guarantee a well-trained labor pool than is recruitment from the outside.

New technology, such as telecommunications and interactive video, can greatly expand educational opportunities for all levels of providers in rural communities. Teleconferences by satellite bring the latest in health care information and training to rural providers. Computer-assisted learning, such as interactive video, can be used alone or in combination with didactic and clinical programs based out of educational institutions to allow rural providers opportunities to further their educations and update their knowledge and skills. However, more needs to be done to ensure that the content of educational programs reflects the needs and realities of the rural environment.

Problems Encountered in
Development and Provision of Services

Barriers in the Physical Environment

In rural areas, distance and the costs of services can be major barriers to long-term care service delivery. Distance is one of the more formidable obstacles to the delivery of in-home services. For persons residing a considerable distance from others needing similar forms of assistance, service delivery can be prohibitively costly and impractical. Rough terrain, poor roads, and inclement weather can pose additional problems for in-home providers and make service costs extremely high.

Financing Care

Financing in-home service delivery in both rural and urban communities is difficult. This is largely the result of our reimbursement systems, which have a pervasive institutional bias. Even when financing is available, such as through Medicaid or Title III, reimbursement rates may be so low that providers will not accept contracts to provide services, fearing they will lose money. There has also been a history of inequitable reimbursement for rural providers. Although some of these inequities are starting to be addressed, rural areas may still have difficulty because of the higher costs of providing in-home services in areas with low population density.

Rural elderly are also less likely than their urban counterparts to have the financial ability to purchase services. According to the Center on Budget and Policy Priorities, poverty occurs as frequently in rural areas as in inner cities. Approximately 16% of rural elderly live on incomes below the poverty level (U.S. Bureau of the Census, 1981) and many more have income levels that preclude the purchase of long-term care services for more than a few days or weeks.

For rural minority elderly, the picture is even more bleak. In 1987, the poverty rate for black elderly in rural areas was 46.5%, compared with 29.2% for black elderly in the central cities. For black elderly women living alone in nonmetropolitan communities, the poverty rate was 79.9% (Bane, 1991). For elderly Native Americans and Hispanics, poverty rates are often higher.

At the rural level, where resources of all types tend to be more scarce, separation of health and social services can drive up costs and can result in unnecessary duplication or gaps in services. Maintenance of separate administrative structures, competition for scarce human resources, and fragmentation of services do not serve older persons' or the community's best interests.

Diversity of Rural Populations

The differences among the individuals who make up rural elderly populations are marked. They differ in ethnic and cultural backgrounds, lifestyles, risk factors, and the personal, economic, and environmental resources available to them. Therefore, there can be no one design for a rural home care delivery system.

The multicultural complexion of this country is clearly manifest in our rural communities and poses both problems and potentials for rural providers. Rural communities are often enclaves of ethnically distinct groups. Although ethnic minority populations can be more easily recognized, it is often forgotten that rural communities may also have very distinct European groups. There are communities where ancestral ties of the residents are linked very closely to Germany, Russia, Ireland, Sweden, Poland, or any number of other countries. Although there is a tendency in the United States to lump these groups together as a single "European" culture, these populations are different from one another. How much their differences in worldviews and social values still carry over in rural enclaves of the United States has received very little attention.

Ethnic minorities also constitute a significant proportion of rural elderly residents. They tend to be poorer, have more health problems, have less adequate housing, and have more difficulty accessing, and possibly less willingness to access, needed services. Rural Native Americans are more than twice as likely as whites to be poor, to be unemployed, and to lack sanitation facilities in their homes (Rhoades, Reyes, & Buzzard, 1987). African American elderly in the rural South rank far below their white counterparts on most economic, housing, and health indicators. Therefore, rural providers must be cognizant of cultural differences as well as equipped to deal with major social, structural, and organizational barriers to home care.

Attitudes and Values

The attitudes and values of rural elderly may create difficulties in the acceptance and provision of in-home services, particularly supportive services. Many rural elderly strongly adhere to a philosophy of self-care and self-reliance. They are not likely to turn to the formal system until their capacities for self-care are seriously threatened or completely exhausted. Even under these circumstances, elders differ in their responses. High suicide rates, particularly among white males faced with incapacitating conditions, illustrate the fear and revulsion many elderly feel about dependency.

Availability of an Adequately Prepared Labor Force

There are ample data that show a smaller proportion of professional health and social services workers in rural than in urban areas. Nurses, therapists, social workers, and in-home support workers are the backbone of the home care system in this country and are in short supply in most rural communities.

The shortage of nurses nationwide has been the focus of numerous studies (U.S. Department of Health and Human Services, 1988a). In recent years, there has been a decrease in the number of nurses working in rural areas (Office of Technology Assessment, 1990). However, it is unclear whether this decrease is a result of a decrease in demand or less interest on the part of nurses to work in rural areas. Interestingly, rural RNs are less likely than urban RNs to be employed in nursing (77% versus 81% in 1988) (Office of Technology Assessment, 1990). A study in 1984 also showed that 14% of rural RNs commuted to urban areas to work, whereas only 2% of urban RNs commuted to rural practice sites (U.S. Department of Health and Human Services, 1988b). This would suggest that higher salary levels and/or more favorable working conditions may be enticing rural nurses to practice in urban areas. On the other hand, the closure of many rural hospitals may leave rural nurses with few other opportunities for employment.

A lower proportion of allied health professionals in rural communities, particularly physical therapists and occupational therapists, has been well documented (Institute of Medicine, 1989). The short supply of PTs and OTs nationally contributes to these differences, but there is also a question of whether the small population bases and lower patient volume of rural areas would support employment of these personnel. It is also unclear whether the lack of PTs and OTs means lack of access to these services in rural communities or whether the services are provided by other health professionals.

There exists very little information on the availability of ancillary health and in-home service workers in rural America. Although providers and residents of rural areas often indicate they have difficulty finding and retaining this level of worker, it is unclear whether the problem is more serious than in urban communities. Poor wages, very difficult and sometimes onerous tasks, and little opportunity for advancement contribute to difficulty in recruiting and retaining these workers. On the other hand, fewer job opportunities in rural communities may result in a greater availability of workers and a higher worker retention rate. This is an area that needs further study.

Program Needs

Information on Needs and Resources

Information on the needs of community residents and the resources for meeting those needs is critical to a rational and efficient planning process. A number of recent mandates from the federal level are moving us closer to the information needed to plan services and allocate resources effectively and efficiently. The implementation nationally of a standardized assessment instrument for all nursing home residents is, for the first time, providing us information on the characteristics of persons entering and residing in nursing homes. A standardized assessment is also being implemented for use with all Medicare beneficiaries being dismissed from hospitals. This will add another piece to the puzzle of long-term care needs among the elderly.

Computerized shared information systems are needed for rational planning and policy decisions at local, state, and national levels. Concerns regarding confidentiality and unintended uses of information have hampered the development of such systems. Although considerable information is gathered by a variety of service providers, there is little sharing of information. Neither is there any uniformity of data categories nor are measurement criteria for quantifying health and functional status standardized among providers.

Establishment of computerized service information systems, containing data on available community services, eligibility criteria, waiting lists, and the like, is also an important step in the development of a community long-term care system. Such systems can facilitate linkage of clients with services and timely recognition of gaps or inadequacies in services, and can provide the quantitative information on service availability needed for policy and planning endeavors.

Financing

Home health care is the most commonly reimbursed form of home care, but reimbursement is limited to persons with relatively acute conditions. Funding for long-term health or supportive services, such as monitoring of chronic conditions, housekeeping, chore services, and personal care, is far more limited and less uniform across geographic areas.

Many bills are now under consideration in Congress that would support a national health care program. It is imperative that national health care and long-term care, both in-home and institutional, be combined into one package in order to avoid the fragmentation of the past and the relegation of home care to the back burner of the care system. Combined health and long-term care programs will allow the development of a more comprehensive continuum of services and reduce the chance of persons being passed inappropriately from one system to another to cut costs in one sector while driving up costs in another.

Professional and Ancillary Human Resources

Human and other resource needs must be carefully and objectively assessed. The concept of specialization and fragmentation of tasks does not work well in rural communities, where trained providers are at a premium. Multiskilled generalists are valuable assets to these communities. As local communities and states seek or develop funding sources for services, they need to break out of traditional service mode categories and develop service approaches most efficient for their needs.

Lack of Complementary Community-Based Services

If a maximum number of older people are to be maintained in independent living settings, community-based services are needed to complement and support in-home services. Services such as adult day care centers, day hospitals, assisted housing, and out-of-home respite services have proven to be cost-effective adjuncts or alternatives to in-home services. However, a critical mass of clients is necessary to make these services financially viable, and finding an adequate and interested client base is not always easy.

Getting residents to services can pose problems in rural communities. Formal transportation systems, if they even exist, are notoriously inadequate in most areas of the United States, with rural areas being the worst. Adequate transportation systems are costly, but they may be far less costly, in monetary and personal terms, than continuing the trend of institutionalizing our disabled older citizens.

Although most older people like to stay in their own homes, many reach a point where this is no longer a feasible alternative. They often find that an institutional setting is the only other available alternative. Housing designed to optimize independence of disabled persons and to provide readily available services can keep older persons out of institutions and reduce the strain on scarce community resources. Housing located in close proximity to basic commercial, social, and health services can allay or at least delay the need for in-home supportive services and for transportation. If in-home services are needed, they can be provided more regularly, effectively, and cost-efficiently if service recipients reside in close proximity.

Core Components of Successful Programs

In this chapter, the concept of a program has focused on a coordinated, comprehensive system of care that may be one program or a number of formally linked programs focused on the same goals. From this perspective, a successful in-home care program should have the elements described below.

Assessment and service planning. Standardized assessment tools provide information to guide service planning, monitor needed changes in service plans, and provide objective data for monitoring the effect of services on expected client outcomes. Combined with standardized formats for written service plans, this assessment and service planning process facilitates an appropriate distribution of resources, as well as provides a written paper path to ensure provider and program accountability.

Strategies for follow-up and plan revision. A written protocol for regular reassessment of clients' needs and a revision of services plans to meet changing needs are vital. These elements require a commitment to individualized care planning, based on objectively assessed needs, and a willingness to offer service packages to meet needs rather than provide services based solely on existing funding streams.

Client-provider partnership in the planning and provision of services. Involvement of the client—or the client's family, if the client is not capable—in the design and strategy for implementing the plan of care is crucial. The need for long-term care does not negate the rights of individuals to make decisions about their lives. Involvement in service planning gives clients the right to accept or refuse needed services and have a say in how those services are to be provided. This not only increases the likelihood that a plan of care will be fully implemented and effective, but also creates a process for making the system more consumer sensitive.

Quality assurance. Quality assurance should be an integral, ongoing part of any service program. It is no longer enough simply to say that a program is "doing great things." Resources are too scarce for funding to be expended on services or programs that have relatively minor or no measurable effects on client outcomes.

Integration of acute and chronic care services. Coordination or integration of health and social services is necessary to ensure that appropriate care is provided without unnecessary duplication or gaps in services. This may be accomplished through formal coordination agreements, case management, or integration of acute and chronic care services under a single administrative and payment structure, with procedures for ensuring appropriate levels of care across all sectors. The latter is the ideal approach, but the most difficult to implement. In the future, national health plans that incorporate long-term care services may make the integration of services the rule, rather than the exception.

Adequately and appropriately trained staff. Successful programs have a commitment to hiring well-trained staff or providing the needed training. They also make available and require staff participation in ongoing educational activities designed to keep their knowledge and skills current. Along with training goes the requirement that job responsibilities be commensurate with training. This is an obligation to clients and an important service to staff.

Adequate salary structures. Salaries should be competitive and should reflect the responsibilities of the persons receiving them. The fact that staff can sometimes be attracted at low wages in rural areas is not an excuse for perpetuating the employment inequities associated with rural residence. Rural providers must receive adequate and competitive salaries and benefits if high-quality, well-trained workers are to be attracted to and remain in rural areas.

Administrators need to be creative in integrating and managing a variety of funding streams, providing data to support client acuity and staffing needs, and lobbying local and state policy makers for the resources to meet these needs adequately. Recruitment and retention of dedicated, well-prepared professionals and ancillary workers mandates that they receive salaries and benefits that are comparable with those received by persons in similar positions in other sectors of the state.

Financial viability. In order to provide continuous, reliable, high-quality services, a program must maintain financial viability. For a program offering a broad spectrum of in-home long-term care and acute care services, this means soliciting and managing monies from diverse sources and negotiating myriad eligibility and reporting requirements.

Leadership. Developing a long-term care program that successfully integrates acute and chronic care services takes leadership. It requires a person or persons who can recognize the needs and have the vision and courage to make changes that address those needs in effective ways. It requires leaders who can clearly articulate their vision and gain the trust and support of others.

A supportive community environment increases the chances that significant change can be instituted and that it will succeed. A program has a chance of success where people are willing to take risks, to try new approaches, and to pay the price necessary to meet the health and long-term care needs of the community.

Research Issues

The following questions arise from some of the issues identified in this chapter as needing additional study:

1. What are the health and functional characteristics of the rural elderly, and how are these characteristics affected by factors such as ethnic diversity, geographic residence, economic status, and resource availability?
2. What are the characteristics of rural elderly that best predict need for and beneficial outcomes from provision of in-home long-term care services?

3. What are the current patterns of service availability and access in rural communities, and how do community and resident characteristics influence these patterns?

4. What influence do different reimbursement systems have on access to services and client outcomes in rural communities?

5. What are the professional and ancillary human resource needs in rural communities today, and what can be done to ensure better availability of needed providers?

6. How effective are our current service approaches in rural areas, and what models of services and service provision work best in rural communities?

Conclusions

There are differences in the health and long-term care needs of urban and rural residents and in available resources to meet these needs. In spite of numerous studies over the past three decades, we still have much to learn about the nature and extent of these differences and how our services systems should be organized to respond effectively to the differences.

Even with this knowledge, the reorganization of service systems will not be easy. The separation of acute and long-term care systems poses an insidious and recalcitrant barrier to the development of a true continuum of care for older Americans. This has occurred, in large part, because of the way in which reimbursement systems have evolved in this country. Significant improvements will take place only when providers and community residents are willing either to integrate existing funding streams creatively or to redesign funding and delivery approaches completely for acute and long-term care services.

Effective reform of our health and long-term care systems requires leaders who recognize the need for change and have the vision and courage to implement the structural and organizational changes necessary to serve older persons better. These changes also will require a significant commitment on the part of community residents. Needed change is likely to mean both financial commitment and some difficult choices in the services to be provided.

The home care service system in the United States, whether in rural or urban communities, does not adequately meet the needs of older Americans. Changes must ultimately be made at the national level to allocate adequate financing for home care services and allow communities the flexibility to design systems of care that will best meet the needs and preferences of their populations. For the near future it is likely that states and local communities will have to bear the burden of making necessary changes, in spite of the federal reimbursement and regulatory structure. Ultimately it will be the battles fought and won by states and the creative energy and pressures from those states that will change our national health and home care system.

12

Mental Health Services for
the Elderly in Rural America

SHARE DeCROIX BANE
ELOISE RATHBONE-McCUAN
JAMES M. GALLIHER

The relationship between physical and emotional health has come under increasing investigation as popular writers have related their own personal stories of increased physical well-being as a result of improving their emotional states. Sports heroes relate their strategies for improving their performance through mental exercises and maintaining a positive emotional state. These are examples of the increasing acceptance of the interrelationship of physical and emotional well-being.

The elderly face increasing physical limitations as well as increasing losses as they grow older. Far more attention has been paid to the physical limitations than to mental and emotional components. The field of mental health itself is comparatively young as a discipline, limiting the understanding of what this discipline has to offer the elderly. Until recently, mental health practitioners have not focused much attention on the elderly. The prevailing schools of psychological treatment were discouraging in their view of the elderly client. At the same time, the current population of elderly are not inclined to understand mental health treatment as a service that is relevant to their needs. For many, the image of "crazy" people in dark and dreary institutions is the extent of their knowledge of mental health. Against this backdrop, a growing number of service providers are trying to introduce a range of mental health services, from preventive services such as telephone re-assurance and support groups that assist in adjustment and a positive sense of well-being to psychiatric assessments and drug therapy.

This chapter presents a current picture of mental health services for the rural elderly, a topic that has received little attention. Mental health services are part of a continuum of care needed by both rural and urban elderly. For many years service availability in rural areas has been thought to be far less than in urban areas. Original data presented in this chapter compare the reported availability in rural and mixed regional areas serviced by the national network of Area Agencies on Aging (AAAs). Although some services are more readily available in rural areas than expected, there is still a national need to press for the development of additional rural mental health services for the aged.

Individual and Environmental Factors Affecting Rural Elderly

In this section we investigate psychological, social, and environmental factors contributing to the mental health of rural elderly. A personal sense of well-being is central to good mental health status in the later stages of the life cycle. In their study of the subjective well-being of rural elderly, Meddin and Vaux (1988) consider the social perspective, consisting of patterns of work, family life, and general social integration, as well as the personality perspective, consisting of life goals and personal success, to interact with the social environment. On the other hand, the rural environmental deficits faced by many older persons play into understanding the well-being of both the individual rural elder and the rural elderly in general.

Factors such as the out-migration of younger people, the farm crisis, and rural hospital closures all affect the economic and social climate of the community as well as what formal services and informal support systems are available. The transactional framework of environmental stress, one that places the human being in continuous interaction with the environment, described by Scheidt and Norris-Baker (1990), offers an interactive perspective of micro and macro stress levels among this population. Health status, for example, directly influences the continuing ability of the person to manage daily living and sustain a satisfactory level of well-being. In a significant number of rural environments, despite their geographic, economic, and/or cultural variations, lifestyle and poverty interact with larger systemic issues of access to formal resources.

The meaning of place, a person's history with the community and home, is also an important intrapersonal dimension affected by environmental conditions. The daily lives of the rural elderly are influenced by economic and social forces that leave them with shrinking supportive resources. Although adaptive compensation, such as redefining a stressful situation to establish positive meaning of social isolation, is a requirement for successful coping in later life (Rathbone-McCuan & Bricker-Jenkins, 1992), the control processes employed by the elderly person may not be sufficient to offset environmental resource depletion.

In optimal circumstances rural elderly persons have informal supports and formal resources available to assist in monitoring the social, emotional, and physical impact of normal aging crises (Coward & Cutler, 1989). Family, friends, neighbors, and other persons assist during illness, provide care to buffer grief and bereavement, and unite against the trauma of residential dislocation. Personalized outreach and individual, family, or group counseling is available to supplement intrapersonal and social network efforts if these personal resources are insufficient to prevent persistent or deteriorating problems of anxiety or situational depression. Unfortunately, the availability of this support is the exception rather than the norm in many communities.

There are other subgroups of rural elderly with acute and chronic mental conditions. Acute psychiatric episodes may require that elderly individuals be taken to a general regional hospital to be seen at either an outpatient clinic or emergency room. The data gathered by Blixen and Lion (1991) in an urban area confirm that elderly do use general hospital outpatient clinics and emergency rooms for acute care needs. Urban areas have more settings with diverse resources to serve geriatric cases. For the rural elderly, geographic and social isolation may delay problem identification and access to appropriate professional help. Once an elder has reached a local or regional rural hospital, restricted policies may preclude his or her admission. If admission to a psychiatric unit is approved, there is little chance that specialized geriatric care will be available.

Buckwalter (1991) concludes, "Little is known about the chronically mentally ill elderly (CMIE) in rural areas, in part because of the lack of services designed to identify and treat community-dwelling rural elderly with long-term mental illness" (p. 216). Blazer (1989b) argues that the increasing percentage of older adults indicates an increased need for epidemiological study. Mental health outreach programs targeting the rural elderly are underdeveloped, and few have been evaluated for service benefits (Buckwalter, McLearan, Mitchell, & Andrews, 1988). Without a means of screening for high-risk conditions or a source of community referral, those with chronic mental illness may be at increased risk. Those with Alzheimer's disease and others with affective disorders (classified by the DSM-III-R to include bipolar disorder, major depression, dysthymic disorder, and atypical depression; Blazer, 1989a) are at risk of institutionalization. Perhaps state hospitals that are experiencing an increased geriatric patient care load (Moak & Fisher, 1991) are assuming a disproportional long-term custodial care function for these rural chronically mentally ill aged.

Status of Rural Mental Health Services

The availability, accessibility, and acceptability of mental health services in rural areas are inadequate. Using these concepts to describe the status of rural mental health services, Human and Watson (1991) note that mental health professionals are concentrated in urban centers and that almost 40% of psychiatrists and psychologists in nonmetropolitan areas are located in rural hospitals. Rural hospitals typically offer a narrower range of services compared with urban centers, which limits the types of services available. Accessibility to mental health services is limited by geographic distance and travel time, the absence of public transportation, limited mental health service outreach, and problems of service reimbursement and program financing (Carscaddon, George, & Wells, 1990; Hargrove & Melton, 1987; Sommers, 1989). Rural residents often find mental health services incompatible with individual, family, and community values because purported rural values support private rather than public means of personal problem solving, and there is a lack of information about emotional and psychiatric care needs. Sources of mental health services in rural areas are often limited to community mental health centers, state hospitals, geographically scattered private mental health practitioners, physicians, and clergy.

Rural private mental health practitioners often have caseloads of poor clients without adequate insurance, thus making services unaffordable to the rural poor. In addition to the lack of a financial base for services, other rural community characteristics confront these practitioners. They may experience difficulties maintaining confidentiality in rural areas; health, social, vocational, industrial, and educational counseling services often overlap, because social networks are very familiar (Spiegel, 1990). Private physicians may be a major source of "patient counseling," especially if they have well-established local practices. On the other hand, Mechanic (1992) takes issue with patients seeking mental health support from physicians who are neither well connected to the mental health system nor well trained and knowledgeable about the use of psychotropic medications and other issues of polypharmacy. They often lack the clinical background and time to provide verbal therapy.

Murray and Keller (1991) note, "In our view, it seems reasonable to conclude that rural populations present substantial rates of psychopathology. It may, however, be overly simplistic and misleading to continually compare rural and urban populations in this regard" (p. 222). Although epidemiological studies are key to understanding risk factors for mental illness and targeting prevention efforts (Blazer et al., 1985; Wagenfeld, Goldsmith, Stiles, & Manderscheid, 1988), mental health centers often proceed to develop services without adequate data.

An example of a need to provide services without adequate information was the demand made on rural mental health centers to provide crisis intervention services for individuals affected by farm failures and foreclosures. The economic and social stresses rural communities faced in the 1980s produced communitywide economic and social stress that disrupted farm families as well as families living in rural towns dependent upon the local farm economy (Fitchen, 1991; Heffernan & Heffernan, 1986; Mermelstein & Sundet, 1986). Rural mental health centers lacked data about the risk characteristics of farm families, yet support services were quickly developed through informal social network structures. In spite of a lack of data, formal mental health services coordinated outreach efforts with the community (Stuve, Beeson, & Hartig, 1989).

In a recent critique of the current status of rural mental health services to the elderly, Rathbone-McCuan (1993) comments that several factors occurring during the 1980s reduced the capacity of community mental health centers to target services to special at-risk populations such as the elderly. The responsibility for federal leadership in public mental health planning lessened. Federal contributions to financing these services were decreased during the 1980s. The transfer of authority from federal- to state-level control helped shift the mandate of community mental health centers from community education and broad outreach efforts to groups such as children and the elderly. Subsequently emphasis turned to providing case management services for the chronically mentally ill.

There are major cracks in many urban and rural mental health service systems (Tausig, 1986). These gaps result in reduced outreach across at-risk groups, greater concentration of in-office-based service delivery, and restricted coordination among mental health, health, and social service resources (Mechanic, 1992). Also, there are fewer clinical specialists trained to target at-risk groups, greater effort is made to offer services to paying clients, and general confusion now exists in the public mental health mission. Major changes are needed in rural mental health programs to improve the accessibility, availability, and acceptability of mental health services to rural elderly facing special social, economic, and environmental risk factors.

State and Local Service Initiatives
for Rural Aging Mental Health

Creative alternatives have been developed in rural communities. Often programs combine various service sectors, such as community mental health facilities and Area Agencies on Aging. These interorganizational working relationships typically develop over time, and their maintenance may be complex and difficult (Lebowitz, Light, & Baily, 1987). When specialized mental health services are not available there are additional resource deficit stressors placed on the formal and informal support networks in rural communities and throughout regional areas.

Because there was limited information available on mental health services for older rural residents, late in 1989 the National Resource Center for Rural Elderly (NRCRE) collected information from state units on aging (SUAs) regarding their mental health efforts for rural elders ("Mental Health," 1990). The information gathered by NRCRE staff indicated that at the state level there was an awareness that rural elderly have mental health needs. For the most part, however, meeting these needs has not been identified as a state-level priority. Although there are not many programs addressing the problem of mental health service delivery in rural areas, the programs that do so are quite varied. Generally this programming exists in one or two service delivery areas within a state and is a coordinated effort involving a mental health provider, a health care provider, and extension services. It is clear that coordination among service delivery agencies is essential, but it is also essential to involve the community as a whole. A review of the information from SUAs indicates that the following programmatic characteristics seem to add to the successful delivery of services:

1. A written interorganizational commitment to provide cooperative service delivery facilitates the resource commitments of all the involved agencies and helps clarify the separate and coordinated/shared care responsibilities.
2. Case management models need to be tailored to the target population and must fit the capacities of the local service network.
3. Coalitions should be formed to cluster resources together to meet the needs of multiple underserved adult populations who are at risk of institutionalization. One of the most effective multiclient efforts seems to be for the combined service needs of the developmentally disabled adult population and older citizens.
4. Mental health agencies need not be the lead service agencies providing all services, but they must be drawn into an active leadership position for planning and monitoring service delivery.
5. An increasing amount of the mental health services that are being provided to the aged need to include attention to the problems of alcoholism and prescription drug abuse.
6. Creative use of communication technology can reduce the impact of distance between clients and professional service providers.
7. Education of the community about services in a manner that is consumer friendly is essential.

The programs described below exemplify these program characteristics and serve as models for reaching the rural elderly with better mental health services.

The Ohio Department on Aging developed an integrated social service model in a rural area. The intents of the project were to ensure that mental health needs of older persons were addressed and to provide a better coordinated case management system. Case management services were very useful in drawing together the formal and informal networks necessary to meet the health, social, and mental health needs of clients.

The Indiana Department of Human Services, Division of Aging Services, developed a program called CHOICE (Community and Home Options to Institutional Care for Elderly and Disabled). The initial program focused on providing support to the physically frail elderly. However, as more emotional and psychiatric problems were identified that produced disability and risks of institutionalization, the services expanded to serve mental health needs.

The Building Ties program was begun by the Michigan Office of Services to the Aging in 1985 with an Administration on Aging grant and is now state funded. Community mental health boards throughout the state participated with the SUA in the project, which sought to improve existing mental health services for the elderly. In many areas new services were developed based on the determined need. The community mental health boards in the program are required to cooperate with local aging offices and must provide mental health services in nontraditional sites, such as homes. Michigan SUA reported excellent interagency cooperation, improvement, and expansion of services.

The Oregon Senior Services Division initiated pilot programs addressing the mental health needs of the elderly, particularly those in rural areas. The goals of the Senior Mental Health project were to enhance local mental health, alcohol, and drug services; to evaluate existing services; to identify gaps in services; and to generate funding.

Staff of mental health service agencies from several states have noted the possible value of using telecommunications as a vehicle to improve outreach to elderly who lack access. As the availability of telecommunications has become widespread in many rural areas, many creative uses have been found to benefit the elderly. One such program was developed by the Eastern Oregon Human Services Consortium in La Grande. This program has grown rapidly and now delivers counseling services to 13 sparsely populated counties through the use of psychiatrists at the Oregon Health Sciences Center. This program uses two-way interactive satellite television and is used for consultation with rural primary care physicians and mental health professionals four hours each week. Satellite television reception studios set up at high schools, hospitals, and community colleges in 7 rural counties are the sites for consultation. Mental health professionals at the Eastern Oregon Psychiatric Center in Pendleton are available via telecommunications to provide crisis and case management. To address the training needs of rural professionals, as well as the development of more professionals, the consortium is developing a distance education program for mental health associates.

Two programs developed on a grassroots level that have been in existence for several years and have proven quite successful are the Mental Health Services of the Rural Elderly Outreach Program in Cedar

Rapids, Iowa, and the Spokane Community Mental Health Center Elderly Services, in Spokane, Washington. There has been considerable evaluation of these programs and there is a substantial body of descriptive information available on them.

The Spokane Community Mental Health Center Elderly Services is a well-developed model. In 1978 only 4% of the agency's active clients were 60 years of age and older; in January 1989 there had been an increase to 21% (Raschko, 1990). This program is composed of telephone information and referral, multidisciplinary in-home evaluation, treatment, and case management. The program has established a gatekeeper system that includes meter readers, bank personnel, county assessors, postal carriers, and telephone company personnel. This system accounts for 4 of every 10 admissions to the in-home case management component. This program is not only successful in providing mental health services but has been conscientious in evaluating the program and serving as a resource to others in order to duplicate the program.

Abbe Center for Community Mental Health of Cedar Rapids, Iowa, in cooperation with the Heritage Agency on Aging, developed an outreach program to serve rural elderly. The program provides on-site psychosocial screening in elderly clinics, churches, and other community settings. Many referrals are made through the more than 500 persons trained as gatekeepers, who help locate and keep track of high-risk elderly.

A multidisciplinary team consisting of a psychiatrist, a nurse, a nurse practitioner, and a social worker conducts in-home mental health assessments. This team also develops treatment plans for patients with psychiatric diagnoses and provides follow-up. This program was initially funded through grants, but it now operates on a fee-for-service basis. The program has been very successful, to the point of needing to limit the number of clients that it can accommodate and serving as a model for replication.

State-level initiatives, especially those that create and maintain cooperative planning and funding between units on aging and departments of mental health, are encouraging necessary steps to better services for the rural elderly. For the rural elderly, the provision of services at the local and regional level will determine the tangible services that are available, accessible, and acceptable. It is imperative that there be cooperation of agencies on federal, state, and local levels if we are to address the barriers to providing services. Linkages among mental health, health, and other aging service providers are a key in any successful program. At the same time, given that we don't know enough about what works, it is important to encourage investigation and evaluation. It is also important to demystify mental health care and educate elders, caregivers, and service providers on mental health issues and services. The bottom line, however, is that for rural service delivery, it is essential to make the program accessible to the rural client. The client must be brought to the service or the service to the client, as demonstrated by the models described above.

Survey of Need and Availability of Mental Health Services

To understand better the rural mental health services available to the elderly, the National Resource Center for Rural Elderly, with assistance from the Center on Rural Elderly, conducted a national survey of need and availability of mental health services. The survey was sent in the spring of 1992 to the executive directors of 615 Area Agencies on Aging. After six weeks, 429 completed and usable surveys had been returned, for a response rate of 70%.

The purpose of the survey was to gather information related to the need, availability, and funding of selected mental health services and programs in AAA planning and service areas (PSAs). The discussion and results that follow are based upon surveys received from rural ($n = 201$) and mixed ($n = 181$) AAAs. *Mixed* AAAs are those in which the planning service areas contain rural, urban, and suburban counties. The designation of a given PSA as urban, rural, or suburban was made by each AAA and specified on the returned survey instrument.

Description of AAAs

How do rural and mixed PSAs compare on selected demographic characteristics? In rural PSAs, the average number of counties served is 5.70; the number is 5.04 in mixed AAAs. The average size of the PSA is 2,954 square miles for rural AAAs and 2,533 for mixed AAAs. Although not much different in terms of numbers of counties served, the rural AAAs have planning service areas approximately 16.6% larger than those of mixed AAAs. The rural AAAs report having to travel an average of 86.91 miles and 3 hours, 4 minutes, to reach their most remote clients; those figures for mixed AAAs are 80.22 miles and 2 hours, 30 minutes. Reaching the most remote clients takes about 21.6% more time for rural AAAs than for mixed AAAs.

Availability of Mental Health Services

The analysis examined availability of what NRCRE had identified from a 1989 state unit inquiry to be the range of potential mental health services that agencies might conceive as part of a mental health care continuum for the elderly. Availability was noted for the following services: adult day care, Alzheimer's support groups, grief/widow support groups, counseling, respite care, telephone reassurance, transportation to mental health services, and visiting in the home/residence. Services more traditionally defined as "mental health" to be checked as available were as follows: advocacy, assessment/screening, education /training, information and referral, and outreach.

The summary data on service availability for rural and mixed PSAs are presented in Table 12.1; these data suggest three major observations. First, of the 14 selected services presented, all are reported available in more than 62% of rural PSAs; grief support is the least available mental health service (62.7%), and telephone reassurance is the most available service (89.6%). Second, 13 of these 14 mental health services are less likely to be available in rural areas compared with mixed areas. Some of these percentage differences between rural and mixed areas are quite small; mental health screening services are available in 88.1% and 89.0% of rural and mixed PSAs, respectively, a difference of about 1%. On the other hand, some differences are glaring; grief support services are available in 86.2% of mixed AAAs, whereas that figure drops to 62.7% for rural PSAs, a difference of 23.5%. Overall, these differences average 9.2% across the 14 mental health services listed. Third, the reported availability of these basic mental health services, especially in rural areas, appears better than generally assumed.

The question referred to availability anywhere within the PSA. It must be kept in mind that a service can be available in one county within a PSA and not in the other counties. The survey also did not inquire as to the *extent* to which these services are available. For example, respite may be available in one county of the PSA and not available in other counties. Even within one county, the respite service may be available only on a limited basis. Moreover, the current data do not document the extent to which an available service is meeting the need for that service in either rural or mixed areas. There was no attempt to determine the

Table 12.1 Availability of Mental Health Services Within Geographic Planning and Service Areas, as Reported by Area Agencies on Aging, 1992 (in percentages)

Service	Rural PSAs	Mixed PSAs	Total
Telephone reassurance	89.6	88.4	89.0
Mental health screening	88.1	89.0	88.5
Counseling	87.6	94.5	90.8
Alzheimer's support group	85.6	97.2	91.1
Mental health referral	83.6	90.6	86.9
Mental health materials	82.6	90.1	86.1
Respite	81.6	91.2	86.1
Mental health transportation	81.6	87.3	84.3
Mental health education	74.1	82.3	78.0
Visiting in the home	72.1	76.2	74.1
Mental health advocacy	71.6	83.4	77.2
Adult day care	69.7	92.3	80.4
Mental health outreach	64.7	75.1	69.6
Grief support	62.7	86.2	73.8

SOURCE: Based on a national mail survey of Area Agencies on Aging. Results presented reflect completed surveys returned from 201 rural and 181 mixed AAAs.

intersection of (a) extent of need, (b) extent of service availability, and (c) extent to which need is being met by the service. Also, the data do not address the issue of the extent to which these services are explicitly targeted to the elderly and/or to other identified populations within a PSA.

Availability of Community Resources

Related to the availability of mental health services themselves is the availability of community resources that facilitate these services to the elderly. Respondents were asked to indicate whether selected community resources were available within their PSAs. These data, shown in

Table 12.2 Availability of Community Resources That Facilitate Mental Health Services to Elderly Within Geographic Planning and Service Areas, as Reported by Area Agencies on Aging, 1992 (in percentages)

Resource	Rural PSAs	Mixed PSAs	Total
Adult protective service intervention for older person with MH problems	80.5	87.2	83.8
Inpatient psychiatric care resources at a local hospital or MH institution	75.0	91.5	83.0
State/regional MH plan that includes the aged	69.2	73.4	71.3
MH consultation available to health care providers	63.5	66.4	65.0
Ombudsman advocacy for older person with MH problems	60.7	61.6	61.1
State/local funding sufficient to support community MH services	33.3	29.4	31.4
Community service planning group advocating for provision of MH services to the elderly	26.3	44.9	35.0
Trained community volunteers to assist older people with MH problems	13.4	24.7	18.7
Mobile MH team that will travel to patient's home	11.9	30.9	20.9

SOURCE: Based on a national mail survey of Area Agencies on Aging. Results presented reflect completed surveys returned from 201 rural and 181 mixed AAAs.

Table 12.2, suggest three observations. First, for both rural and mixed PSAs, there is considerable variability in the availability of these community resources. Within rural PSAs, these range from 80.5% for adult protective service intervention to only 11.9% for mobile mental health team, the former being 6.8 times more likely to be in place in rural areas than the latter. In mixed areas, this variability is just as great. These resources vary from a high of 91.5% for inpatient psychiatric care to a low of 24.7% for community volunteers trained to assist older persons with mental health problems.

Second, although some differences in resources between rural and mixed PSAs are small (e.g., ombudsman advocacy for older persons with mental health problems), some are striking and point to the relative disadvantage of rural planning service areas. For example, whereas the two resources of community service planning groups advocating for provision of mental health services to the elderly and mobile mental health teams are available within 44.9% and 30.9% of mixed PSAs, respectively, these figures decrease to 26.3% and 11.9% for rural PSAs. Overall, the differences average about 8.5% across the community resources listed, with the rural PSAs lagging behind mixed PSAs. Third, as was true in the discussion on the mental health services themselves, there is a striking similarity in the relative availability of these selected resources from high to low when comparing rural and mixed PSAs. Resources that are generally not available in mixed areas are not likely to be available in rural areas, and vice versa.

Funding for Mental Health Services

The survey also asked respondents to indicate whether their AAAs funded these available services either partially or fully within the PSAs. If funded only partially by the AAAs, these services were funded by other sources as well. These summary data are presented in Table 12.3; they suggest three major observations. First, there is a great deal of variation within both rural and mixed PSAs with respect to the AAAs' funding of mental health services. To illustrate, 68.4% of rural AAAs fund respite programs; that figure drops to only 4.5% for mental health screening. Thus rural AAAs are more than 15 times more likely to fund respite programs (in whole or in part) than they are to fund mental health screening. For mixed AAAs, the high and low figures are 69.6% for respite services and 12.1% for both grief support services and mental health materials. Second, of the 14 services presented, only 5 are reported funded by AAAs in more than 50% of rural PSAs and mixed PSAs. Third, 10 of the 14 mental health services are less likely to be funded by the AAAs in rural areas, compared with AAAs in mixed areas.

One limitation of these data is that they do not specify either the AAA absolute level of funding (e.g., actual dollars per fiscal year) or the relative level of funding (e.g., percentage of budget per fiscal year) for specific types of mental health services and/or mental health services in general. Similarly, the data do not discuss the AAAs' sources of

Table 12.3 Funding for Selected Mental Health Services by AAAs Within Planning and Service Areas, as Reported by Area Agencies on Aging, 1992 (in percentages)

Service	Rural PSAs	Mixed PSAs	Total
Respite	68.4	69.6	69.0
Visiting in the home	61.8	56.9	59.4
Telephone reassurance	60.9	54.0	57.6
Mental health transportation	60.0	58.4	59.2
Adult day care	52.8	63.0	58.2
Alzheimer's support group	31.8	24.4	28.1
Mental health referral	20.3	26.6	23.4
Counseling	17.2	27.2	22.2
Grief support	11.7	12.1	12.0
Mental health outreach	10.3	12.7	11.5
Mental health materials	8.5	12.1	10.2
Mental health advocacy	7.8	16.8	12.5
Mental health education	5.4	13.7	9.6
Mental health screening	4.5	13.5	8.9

SOURCE: Based on a national mail survey of Area Agencies on Aging. Results presented reflect completed surveys returned from 201 rural and 181 mixed AAAs.
NOTE: Funding is provided in whole or part by the AAA within its PSA; that is, the funding is provided only by the AAA or by the AAA and other funders. Percentages shown refer to only those agencies reporting that a given service is available within their PSAs (see Table 12.1).

funding for mental health services; that is, through the "AoA funding stream" or other funding streams. There is also no assessment of how AAA funding of mental health services for the elderly is related to either (a) the availability of services or (b) the actual assessment of mental health needs among elderly populations.

Perceived Importance of Mental Health Services

The survey instrument presented brief descriptions of 19 selected mental health services and asked respondents to evaluate each of these according to their perceived importance for the elderly within their PSAs. These service descriptions and their mean importance scores are presented in Table 12.4. The data suggest three major observations about the importance of these mental health services. First, there is some—although not extensive—variation within both sets of respondents as to how important these selected mental health services are evaluated to be. (Given that respondents selected responses between 1 and 5 to represent their evaluations of the importance of these services, the relatively small variability observed across these items is not surprising.) For example, both groups of respondents view mental health programs targeted toward the elderly as the most important of these services, with mean scale scores of 1.68 (rural) and 1.64 (mixed). Likewise, both groups view the need for more psychiatrists as the least important services, with mean scores of 2.87 (rural) and 3.01 (mixed). Second, despite this observed variation within each group, both groups tend to evaluate each of the listed services as "more" important rather than "less" important. On a 5-point scale (1 being most important need and 5 being least important), all but one of the mean importance scores across both groups of respondents are less than 3.00, the hypothetical midpoint of the 5-point continuum. Third, the two respondent groups show little absolute difference between their collective evaluations of specific services. For their evaluations of mental health outreach for caregiver families, the mean responses are identical at 1.83; for their evaluations of psychological/social programs for congregate living, their responses diverge the most, with mean scores of 2.49 (rural) and 2.28 (mixed). Fourth, the two sets of respondents display considerable similarity in their overall importance rankings of these mental health services (Spearman's rho = .967). This means that both groups concur highly in their views of the relative importance of these mental health services for elderly clients within their PSAs.

Although the data display a high degree of relative congruence at the aggregate level between AAA respondents from rural and mixed PSAs in their evaluations of the importance of selected mental health services, these data are not without their limitations. For example, there is no indication as to why respondents evaluate selected services as more (or less) important. Some services may be more important than others because of their relative low costs (although not necessarily cost-effectiveness). Other unavailable services may be evaluated as important because of their presumed or anticipated benefits. Still other services may not be seen as important because they are simply not currently

Table 12.4 Mean Perceived Importance Scores Given to Mental Health Services and Programs Within Geographic Planning and Service Areas, as Reported by Area Agencies on Aging, 1992

Service	Rural PSAs	Mixed PSAs	Total
MH programs for elderly	1.68	1.64	1.66
Medicare for MH services	1.79	1.77	1.78
Medicaid for MH services	1.81	1.84	1.82
MH outreach for caregiver families	1.83	1.83	1.83
MH staff with aging expertise	1.89	1.71	1.80
Nursing home care for MH patients	1.93	1.91	1.92
MH education for elderly	1.95	1.93	1.94
MH education for caregivers	1.97	1.90	1.94
Intervention resource abuse	2.03	1.90	1.97
Geriatric MH education for providers	2.05	1.96	2.01
MH assessment for elderly	2.07	2.05	2.06
Professional MH consulting for nursing homes	2.15	1.99	2.07
Location of MH services	2.21	2.05	2.14
Drug education for elderly	2.25	2.24	2.30
Drug education for caregiver	2.30	2.28	2.29
MH service referral mechanism	2.41	2.32	2.37
Psychological/social programs for congregate living	2.49	2.28	2.39
Social workers	2.64	2.79	2.71
Psychiatrists	2.87	3.01	2.94

SOURCE: Based on a national mail survey of Area Agencies on Aging. Results presented reflect completed surveys returned from 201 rural and 181 mixed AAAs.
NOTE: The smaller the mean rank score, the greater the perceived importance of the mental health service.

offered within a given PSA. And even for those services that are viewed as extremely important, this question needs to be addressed: For which mental health problems are these services important? Some services may be quite successful for some problems and not successful for others. Clearly, more study needs to be conducted on what specific services are needed to meet specific mental health needs of the elderly in different locations.

Ranking of Mental Health Problems

Apart from the availability, funding, and importance of mental health services, respondents were also asked to rank a number of mental health problems that are generally believed to be associated with aging. Table 12.5 presents the mean ranks and shows a great deal of variation within both sets of AAA respondents as to how they view these mental health problems within their PSAs. Indeed, when it is remembered that respondents ranked these items on a 10-point scale (from 1, *most need,* to 10, *least need*), the mean scale scores suggest that they are able to discriminate readily in their perceptions of the needs associated with these problems. For example, respondents believe that loneliness and depression are the most pressing mental health problems. In rural areas, the mean importance scores are 2.52 and 2.62 for these two problems; for mixed areas, these figures are 3.05 and 2.51. Likewise, respondents believe that personality disorder is the least serious of these mental health problems, with mean scores of 8.84 and 8.83. Second, the two sets of respondents show very little difference in their evaluations of specific problems. For their evaluations of personality disorder, the mean responses are almost identical (8.84 versus 8.83); for their evaluations of loneliness, their responses diverge the most, with mean scores of 2.52 (rural) and 3.05 (mixed). Third, the two sets of respondents display remarkable similarity in their overall ranking of these problems from most to least serious. When the two sets of mean responses given by rural and mixed respondents are ranked and compared, this results in a rank correlation (Spearman's rho) of .976. This means that there is almost perfect agreement (i.e., rho approaches 1.00) between these two sets of respondents' evaluations of these mental health problems and issues. Respondents from rural and mixed AAAs ostensibly are able to differentiate among several types of mental health problems and disorders and to agree in their differentiations. This suggests that there is considerable agreement within the aging network as to which mental health problems among the elderly are in most need of intervention.

Table 12.5 Mean Rank Scale Scores Given to Mental Health Problems of the Elderly Within Geographic Planning and Service Areas, as Reported by Area Agencies on Aging, 1992

Problem	Rural PSAs	Mixed PSAs	Total
Loneliness	2.52	3.05	2.77
Depression	2.62	2.51	2.57
Memory impairment	4.24	4.47	4.35
Anxiety	4.44	4.69	4.56
Grief	4.58	4.65	4.61
Adjustment	5.45	5.28	5.37
Drug misuse	6.69	6.46	6.58
Alcoholism	6.96	6.71	6.83
Paranoia	8.21	8.19	8.20
Personality disorder	8.84	8.83	8.84

SOURCE: Based on a national mail survey of Area Agencies on Aging. Results presented reflect completed surveys returned from 201 rural and 181 mixed AAAs.
NOTE: The lower the mean rank scale score, the greater the perceived need for mental health services for the problem or issue.

One limitation of these findings is the relatively small number of mental health problems evaluated. Owing to time and resource constraints, this reduced the number of mental health "problems" that could be reasonably included in the survey. No attempt was made to randomly sample a subset from all possible mental health problems, even assuming that such a list could be enumerated. In the selection of problems, the approach was to include a representative subset that was presumed to cover the entire range of possible problems from least to most need of intervention. Obviously, the choice of problems selected may have affected these evaluations and the extent to which respondents agreed in their evaluations. Had some of the problems' descriptive labels been reworded or excluded and other descriptions included, this may have influenced the overall results.

Another possible limitation is the actual question wording presented to respondents. The survey instructions asked individuals to evaluate the mental health problems "according to the needs of the elderly." This instruction could have been interpreted in a number of ways by respondents. They could have taken it to refer to the prevalence or incidence of these problems among the elderly; that is, from least to most prevalent or frequent. To others it could have meant the "seriousness" or "severity" or "harmfulness" of these problems to either the elderly experiencing these problems or the community as a whole. To still others it could have meant the ease or difficulty in resolving these problems among the elderly experiencing them. These possible different interpretations may indeed have resulted in different patterns of responses and more (or less) agreement among respondents. Although there may have been a high degree of similarity in how the same respondents evaluate these different properties (namely, need, seriousness, prevalence, and difficulty of resolution) of the mental health problems posed, there is nothing in the data or survey results themselves that would suggest such an observation.

Ranking of Elderly Populations in Need of Mental Health Services

The survey also asked respondents about their perceptions of which elderly populations were in most (and least) need of mental health services. Mean rank scores representing respondents' collective evaluations are given in Table 12.6. Respondents appear quite able to distinguish among these selected elderly populations in terms of their needs for mental health services. The two groups concur that adult protective services clients are in most need and that farm-based elderly are in least need. Indeed, the ranks given to each group's set of evaluations are in close agreement with each other (Spearman's rho = .979).

The last series of questions, including both service priority rankings and narrative explanations of rankings, provided information about what resources directors wanted to see developed within PSAs to improve the quality of mental health care for elderly persons. The presence of more specialized mental health personnel and programs were considered most important by both types of AAAs. General mental health services were not considered adequate to target the most at-risk elderly. Many AAA respondents discussed the lack of Medicare and Medicaid coverage for mental health services as fundamental barriers that must be reduced before there could be any realistic expectations of recruiting and supporting more professional geriatric mental health expertise in the PSA. The three areas where respondents felt that existing mental

Table 12.6 Mean Rank Scale Scores Given to Elderly Populations in Need of Mental Health Services and Programs Within Geographic Public and Service Areas, as Reported by Area Agencies on Aging, 1992

Elderly Population	Rural PSAs	Mixed PSAs	Total
Adult protective services clients	3.34	3.19	3.26
Alzheimer's victims	3.35	3.36	3.36
Homebound	3.56	3.61	3.58
Caregivers	3.98	4.49	4.22
Former mental hospital patients	4.11	3.94	4.02
Widowed women	4.15	4.49	4.32
Widowed men	4.51	4.93	4.71
Homeless	7.19	6.54	6.85
Minority	7.28	7.01	7.14
Farm based	7.67	8.13	7.89

SOURCE: Based on a national mail survey of Area Agencies on Aging. Results presented reflect completed surveys returned from 201 rural and 181 mixed (rural and urban) AAAs.
NOTE: The lower the mean scale score, the greater the perceived need of specified elderly populations for mental health services and programs.

health services could do more for the elderly population were general outreach and education, support groups and counseling for the families of caregivers of frail elderly, and active involvement in cases of elder abuse and neglect in both the community and institutions such as local nursing homes. Concern for increasing the accessibility of existing service resources was expressed and mobile teams or community-based mental health personnel were considered as essential to reach the elderly who either could not or would not seek assistance available in a typical agency setting.

Policy and Research Directions

Rural gerontologists and human service providers continue to struggle with strategies that help focus attention on the needs of those aged persons living in nonmetropolitan areas. There is agreement that research, innovative program expansion, and policy reform must take into account what is unique about growing old and being old in rural America. Mental health needs and programs for rural elderly should be incorporated into the larger health care planning context; however, mental health must also be considered in the larger social services system. Adding a mental health perspective into the social service and health care delivery and financing debate does not mean that it should be excluded from more specialized psychiatric and mental health care areas, but that the latter policy and practice arena is too narrow.

The successful mental health programs operating to serve the rural elderly are ones that are carefully integrated into other community service resources. Resources and expertise are shared and older clients move into and out of services in a monitored flow supported through case management and client advocacy functions. Successful services emphasize physical and psychological accessibility. Although fiscal resources are not abundant, the financial base of program operations is sufficiently stable to keep programs operating with some sense of permanence. This stability has been important in gaining client and provider acceptance affecting service utilization.

In the short term, priority must be given to several issues of mental health concern. First priority must be given to research that helps to clarify further the specific mental health needs of rural elderly in specific catchment and service planning areas. Data that identify the unique problems of rural elderly women and minority rural elders are particularly needed. The means of collecting and analyzing information must be adequate if data are to be used in program planning and policy and legislative change. This should include the perceptions of mental health problems and issues among the rural elderly and how they affect the accessing of services.

A second consideration is to find ways of drawing rural service providers into an ongoing and substantial regional planning process. It is important to know what mental health services can be cost-effectively delivered under a regional model and what resources must be localized. For example, developing the capacity to provide in-home mental health assessments is a very much needed resource for the rural elderly at a local level. On the other hand, more complex and comprehensive neuropsychiatric assessments involving attention to biomedical concerns can best be accomplished in regional facilities where the appropriate interdisciplinary expertise is available.

Third, considerably greater attention must be given to the mental health care needs of those caregivers who are sustaining the psychiatrically ill elderly in the community. There are numerous models of psychoeducation relevant to the chronic mentally ill population that can be adapted to fit issues of illness in later life. Community mental health centers can appropriately assume leadership to test and evaluate such programs in order that core information can be delivered effectively by other service providers having regular contact with the elderly and their caregivers. This information is of great importance to those who deliver protective services or in-home health care to the rural elderly. Geriatric mental health training is also needed in order to build the capacity of volunteers to be of greater assistance to elderly individuals with mental illness in both community and institutional settings. Interdisciplinary training and mentorships in applied settings are needed to increase the availability of trained personnel and to increase understanding.

Fourth, building a better planning mechanism that can effectively integrate mental health and aging services development remains a challenge at both federal and local levels. The rural perspective must be given as much attention as major inner-city areas. The National Institute of Mental Health must be provided with the resources needed to implement the new rural mental health agenda that has been framed, but remains unfunded. Without that national leadership to address the specific issues facing the rural elderly and their mental health needs, there is little chance that broad-based policy reform and service delivery expansion will be developed.

Summary and Conclusions

This chapter has focused on the mental health needs of rural elderly and has discussed specific services that either are available or need to be added into the spectrum of service to the rural aged. Given the national concern with the broad medical care crisis, less rather than more direct attention is now focused on mental health. Meeting the needs of the chronically mentally ill remains the greatest mandate for the public mental health system, yet both rural and urban areas lack sufficient funds to address the complex needs of the most severely impaired and at the same time expand programs to other underserved populations.

In our discussion, we have attempted to summarize what factors contribute to the availability, accessibility, and acceptability of mental health services for the rural aged. Administrators of AAAs in both rural and mixed PSAs see that the general continuum of mental health services could be made more relevant with the addition of specialized staff and targeted programs that address the psychosocial needs of the aged, including those who care for them and suffer mental health risks from the caregiving process.

In the short term, there is a need to clarify further what role health and social services can assume in protecting the mental health status of rural elderly through attention to the processes and events of normal aging that create depression, loneliness, and anxiety. Greater involvement from these service sectors will not eliminate the need for formal and specialized mental health services for the older rural population; however, it may provide a more integrated approach to building a framework for geriatric mental health care planning and service delivery.

Epilogue

JOHN A. KROUT

The purpose of this book is to increase understanding of the provision of a wide range of community-based services to older persons living in rural environments. In order to do this, each of the chapters first presents a brief review of the needs of this population that can be met, at least partially, through community-based services. The chapters are based in reviews of existing research on the needs of the rural elderly for particular services, but they focus on the standard community-based service approaches generally in place to meet needs, alternative strategies that can be adopted to provide each service, and the core elements or building blocks of successful rural programming. To delineate successful approaches, the contributors make suggestions for overcoming the barriers to developing and providing effective community-based services in rural settings. They also identify central research and policy questions that need to be resolved if efforts to meet the needs of older rural populations through various community-based service modes are to be more successful in the future.

The underlying assumption of this book is that, although it has been very difficult at times, the provision of effective community-based services to rural older persons has been and is being done. Thus the emphasis here is not on what cannot be done, but on what can be done. The authors do not, by and large, present step-by-step instructions on "how to do" various community-based services. Providing such detailed information for even one service would require a book in and of itself. It would also do violence to one of the fundamental observations repeated in every chapter—the great variability that characterizes rural populations and areas requires that general programmatic approaches be refined and adapted for each setting.

The need for community- and population-specific program approaches notwithstanding, what generalizations does the information presented in these diverse chapters support? What needs of rural older populations are effectively addressed by various community-based services? What commonalities underlie the provision of community-based services to older rural populations that practitioners, researchers, and policy makers should recognize and respond to? What common themes or threads run through the most appropriate and effective approaches to providing these services? What barriers are most likely to be encountered, and how can they be overcome? What outstanding research questions should be investigated? What policies need to be strengthened, changed, or developed in order to improve the availability and effectiveness of community-based services for older rural persons?

Rural Older Populations

As noted in the introductory chapter and reinforced by contributions to this volume, the need for greater attention to the planning, development, presentation, and funding of community-based services among rural older persons is rooted in many different circumstances. First, we have the characteristics of older rural persons in general. Research has shown that on the whole this population is disadvantaged relative to elders living in other residential settings. Older rural persons have lower incomes and fewer opportunities for income enhancement, reside in older and less adequate housing, experience more health problems and greater levels of impairment in a number of areas, and are more likely to be dependent on private vehicles for transportation because of a lack of transport alternatives. They have lower levels of formal education as well. It has also been suggested that the value and belief systems of rural elders not only may contribute to their need for community-based services, but may decrease their willingness to seek assistance and utilize whatever services might be available. The experiences and life-styles of rural older populations are also noted as important factors that must be considered in the development and provision of community-based services. Thus there is considerable evidence to support the argument that rural community-based services are needed and should be a high priority within the aging services network, but that they cannot simply be scaled-down versions of urban-based programs.

Rural Communities

The characteristics of rural areas and communities compound and magnify the needs of rural older persons and have significant impacts on the ways in which these needs can be met. These characteristics include low population density and size, which affect service provision in many ways, and a lack of economic and other resources to support service development and operation. The factor that probably is mentioned more than any other by the contributors to this volume is service access, generally expressed as a lack of transportation. With large distances between people, many service delivery modes are either impractical or too expensive to work in rural areas. Getting people to services (or vice versa) then becomes a central challenge to rural community-based service providers. This condition actually reinforces the importance of developing adequate *local* community-based services that are easily accessed.

Several chapter authors suggest that transportation policies, programs, and resources do exist at the state and federal levels and are utilized to address the access challenge, but that they are inadequately funded, unduly restrictive, and need to be examined carefully for unintended rural "penalties." The authors argue that this does not have to be the case. As noted, transportation programs can be made more effective and cost-efficient, especially if more resources are provided, not only to pay for vans, tires, and gasoline, but also for the training of agency staff and volunteer boards on how to manage rural transportation systems. Further, as has been noted by at least one set of authors, the transportation problems that plague rural community-based services reflect land-use patterns that have led to the centralization of many services.

A number of the contributors also note another issue that is partly related to population density: the availability and diffusion of service information. They observe that the level of service awareness and understanding of services is low among rural older populations. The solution to this information gap may lie partly in the greater utilization of modern communication technology. On the other hand, authors also argue that the local rural information networks need to be utilized more frequently and effectively, but with care to ensure that the appropriate information is being shared. Although "high-tech" solutions often seem irresistible to policy planners, they may or may not be well accepted by various rural populations. Again, the chapter authors call for greater attention to these alternatives.

The ecology of rural areas (low population density, small population centers, topography) complicates the development and provision of rural community-based services in other ways. Low population densities usually mean greater distances between service providers and clients, and between clients and clients, which in turn can translate into higher overall service costs or a disproportional amount of resources being dedicated to access services. Low population densities discourage the development of services because of a lack of economies of scale. Without a sufficient number of consumers, private providers cannot justify the investment of resources in rural areas. Health services such as hospitals have had difficulty surviving in rural areas, especially when they have had to compete with urban specialists. The result has been lack of service availability across the board in community-based services. Rural areas do not support the number, diversity, and depth of services and service professionals often found in more urban places.

One might argue that in a market economy, this is the way it should be, and that low density/population areas that cannot support the full range of services simply will not have them. Again, chapter authors argue that creativity and flexibility can help some services "stay local." Many examples can be found around the country in the health care field of sustaining a reasonable level of health care in rural areas even as anchor providers such as hospitals scale back services or close. Partnerships with urban hospitals, universities, private physicians, and the like have begun to respond to the crisis in rural health care. The same can be attempted with various community-based services. Of course, we must also recognize that many times needed health and social services simply are not available at all in rural areas.

Difficulties with the economic feasibility of providing community-based services in many rural areas highlight another aspect of those areas that affects community-based services for older persons—the need for economic development in rural America. Without a strong economic base, many rural areas simply lack the economic wherewithal to support needed services. The depopulation of many rural areas has been a consequence of the loss of jobs tied not only to the mechanization of extractive industries but also to the inability of many rural areas to provide the kinds of amenities that attract employers. And with so many new jobs tied to the service sector, population losses deal a double blow to rural areas. Rural out-migration has also been noted as a factor in the depletion of informal and volunteer networks to assist older persons who want to remain in their homes. This issue needs to be seen as one not just of economic development, but of community development. Some rural communities have successfully generated or attracted manufacturing industry; others have benefited from tourism and recreation. A number of the chapter authors point out the need to build strong linkages between the service and private sectors in rural areas.

External Factors

Another observation that reflects sentiments expressed by the contributors is that many factors external to rural areas combine to act as disincentives to service providers working in rural areas and, therefore, to the disadvantage of rural populations. Government reimbursement policies, personnel standards, funding mechanisms and availability, policy emphases and priorities, and program content and targeting, among others, are identified as the culprits. Several authors question the geographic equity in current program funding schemes and suggest that subtle or not-so-subtle biases lead to either inadequate resources or, worse, a type of "benign neglect" of rural needs. These charges are difficult to prove, but they do raise an important question: What constitutes a rural "fair share" of program resources? These concerns highlight some fundamental policy issues. I suggest that part of the problem lies in the perpetuation of "stereotypes" of older rural populations, which only recently have been examined closely. Virtually all of the chapter authors call for a greater infusion of resources for the support of rural community-based services for the elderly, a sentiment with which I would heartily concur. Like service providers in many areas, rural practitioners have seen the number of people in need, the degree of service need, and the time over which care is needed increase.

This is not a uniquely rural phenomenon, but it does have uniquely rural dimensions, and this is the fact that as much as anything needs to be better understood and addressed. Most of the authors do not dwell on this issue; rather, they devote their energies to discussing how, given the resources available, rural community-based services to the elderly can be provided successfully. It is not necessarily a question of asking rural providers to do *more* without additional resources, a practice that has increased over the past two decades as the federal and even state governments have mandated services that local governments must then find a way to fund. Rather, the authors suggest ways to improve what is currently being done.

Elements of Success

This brings us to a very important arena of discussion—the elements that contribute to successful rural community-based programming. Many of these elements likely would apply to service development and provision in nonrural settings as well. The important underlying point made over and over again by the authors is the need to assess how these elements should be constructed or modified to meet the conditions of each rural area and the characteristics, values, and beliefs of the older persons living there. This reflects the need to recognize that diversity characterizes rural America. The inability or unwillingness of service providers and policy makers to recognize and respond appropriately to this diversity is surely one of the most frequent and serious failings affecting rural aging programs. Further, the authors consistently point out that this rural uniqueness and diversity needs to be explicitly accounted for in professional education, training, and technical assistance efforts, and in yardsticks used to evaluate individual and program performance. This has begun to be done to at least some degree in a number of health and social service areas.

Many of the ideas on best practice approaches are based in what I have identified in the introductory chapter and other authors allude to as the "A words": availability, accessibility, appropriateness, acceptability, awareness, affordability, and adequacy. Rural community-based service policies and programs need to be examined in light of how well they achieve each of these conditions for the rural elderly, not the convenience of program staff or bureaucratic accounting or management. Making a service available does not just mean ensuring that it is in place, but that it is provided at times and in places that fit the needs and preferences of the people for whom it truly is intended. A fixed-route transportation system may make a lot of sense given the shortage of rural transport resources, and congregate nutrition or adult day care programs might be offered on a certain schedule in response to the availability of staff or facilities. But if these schedules or the services are not consistent with the needs and preferences of those for whom they are intended, the services will be difficult to justify and will surely fail. Rural community-based services are not like the fabled baseball field in the popular movie *Field of Dreams,* as at least one author notes. Making a service "available" does not necessarily mean those in need of it will be served. Most rural practitioners understand this full well, but find themselves unable to follow through on it because of a lack of resources or because guidelines promulgated by funders require them to provide only certain services in certain ways. This is why many rural community-based practitioners ask for more flexibility in programming.

What are some of the other factors noted by authors as helpful to success? We are constantly reminded to learn and understand the nuances of local communities' cultures and values, and to recognize and utilize existing local support networks. We are reminded that rural people (and communities), even those who seem to be only barely functioning, have pride, strengths, and resources that should be built upon, not bypassed or, even worse, negated or weakened. Building on local resources is likely to be more cost-effective and successful than starting from scratch with new ones. This recognition would seem basic to earning and keeping another important component of program success— the trust of those in need and their families. Sensitivity to rural diversity based on race and ethnicity clearly is as important a consideration as recognizing diversity among rural areas based on other factors.

Finally, as would be expected, all of the authors note the need for greater coordination among providers and between providers and everyone else, and for more attention to private-public partnerships. Although the call for "coordination" sounds like a wornout cliché, it rings as true today as it did 20 years ago, when organizations such as Area Agencies on Aging emerged out of the Older Americans Act and many of the community-based services examined in this book first began to develop. In fact, many circumstances in the aging services network today have led to an even greater need for coordination. The numbers and types of services have grown, funding streams and reimbursement mechanisms and regulations have become more complex, and the "competition" for resources (and clients) has become fierce. All of this has occurred in an era of expanding and increasingly long-lived older populations, shrinking resources, and, for many rural areas, challenges to economic and community survival. Lacking sufficiently large client bases, rural community-based service providers in particular must work with each other to meet the needs of older persons more efficiently. But aiming for more coordination does not mean that more standardization is necessarily a key to better programs. As several contributors note, successful rural programming requires many different service modes and approaches. Flexibility, innovation, and the willingness to try new things are essential.

Research Questions

Many specific research questions are identified in this volume. For every service, the need for much more research on the most basic aspects of its operation in rural circumstances is noted. Very few data are available on the factors related to rural community-based service availability, accessibility, utilization, impact, and effectiveness. The authors note especially the need for program evaluation studies so that successful program model components can be better understood and information on them more widely disseminated. Surveys, case studies, and longitudinal research are all seen as essential. Much emphasis is also placed on the importance of gaining a greater understanding of the variation in needs and effective program responses found in different rural areas. I would like to offer the following as "generic" research questions on rural community-based services for the elderly that are in need of investigation:

1. What is the importance of various factors in explaining residential differences in the availability or distribution of different community-based services?
2. What is the importance of community-based service utilization for residential differences in the health status of older rural populations?
3. What is the importance of various factors in explaining variation in community-based service awareness, acceptance, and utilization among older rural populations?
4. What factors account for residential differences in the relationship between receipt of informal care and the utilization of community-based services?
5. What are the consequences of the availability, accessibility, and utilization (or lack thereof) of various community-based services for rural communities?
6. Are residential differences in health status for "at-risk" older persons (based on race, ethnicity, income, gender, or living situation) related to the availability, accessibility, or utilization of community-based services?

7. What are the core components or essential elements of successful rural community-based service approaches, and how do these differ by residential setting?

8. What is the importance of various barriers, as perceived by older persons and practitioners and in reality, to the availability, accessibility, and utilization of community-based services for rural older persons?

9. What residential differences exist in the components of successful programming and in the training and technical assistance needs of community-based service professionals and volunteers?

It would also seem important to point out that there is not currently in place a uniform set of criteria for the reporting, collection, and analysis of information on community-based services nationally. Thus information from various programs or existing studies available to researchers and policy makers is not comparable. Work toward such a uniform system clearly would be useful for research designs, program development, and policy decisions. For example, questions about rural/urban differences in service availability and cost and the most appropriate ways to address them are difficult to answer with the data currently available.

Policy Issues

I conclude this epilogue with a brief consideration of policy issues. A number of the contributors to this volume argue that policies affecting the expenditure of health and social service dollars have intentionally or unintentionally favored urban areas and shortchanged rural populations and that there is a lack of residential equity in the distribution of services and service professionals. The proof of this bias is found, they say, in the lack of availability of many community-based services in rural communities even though the older persons in these places are relatively disadvantaged and in at least as great or greater need of the services as older persons residing in urban areas. In addition, existing policies include little recognition of the variation found in rural America.

I find such arguments compelling, but caution that they oversimplify the complexity of the situation that leads to disadvantages and deficiencies in rural community-based services for older persons. Policy directions, funding allocations, and program mandates to be sure all can have negative impacts on rural service availability and accessibility, but so can economic and demographic shifts that are largely untouched by policy. Additionally, the data needed to demonstrate with certainty the impacts of past and current policies are lacking. It is important to examine the impacts of existing reimbursement mechanisms, program and funding targeting, education and training programs, and expectations for staff credentials on rural community-based services. As many of the chapter authors observe, it is also important to develop new policies and funding strategies that recognize and support the needs of older rural persons and the uniquely rural responses to these needs.

We often hear about the need to bring greater "equity" to existing policy, program efforts, and expenditures, both among the elderly and for individuals based on age, income, gender, and race. I would urge, as I have done previously, that there is a need for greater equity in service availability and accessibility for older persons living in rural areas. Individuals should not, simply because they live in low-density and low-population areas, be denied access to needed services. But the concept of equity is difficult to define and even more difficult to implement. Can or should very rural populations have available and easily accessible to them every service they may need? Should this be one of the goals of health and human service policy for the elderly? If so, how can this best be done, and how should it be paid for? We can answer, in principle, that complete service equity should be a policy goal and that these services should be made available to all rural elders. Realistically, however, the expense and difficulty of achieving this condition may require compromises. We face difficult decisions on just what the community-based service priorities for older rural populations should be.

It is my hope that the chapters in this book provide information that will help researchers, practitioners, and policy makers work toward developing these priorities and achieving the goal of improved community-based service coverage and quality for rural elders, given the fact that all the resources necessary to achieve this goal will likely never become available. Progress has been made in developing coordinated community-based care systems that identify and respond to the needs of impaired rural elders. We have been more successful in some areas than others (e.g., congregate nutrition programs as opposed to mental health services), and much more work needs to be done. The challenge is clearly here and awaits our continued efforts to meet it.

References

Alliance of Information and Referral Systems. (1983). *National standards for information and referral.* Alexandria, VA: United Way of America.

American Association of Retired Persons. (1990). *Understanding senior housing for the 1990s: An AARP survey of consumer preferences, concerns, and needs.* Washington, DC: Author.

American Association of Retired Persons. (1991a). *A profile of older Americans.* Washington, DC: Author.

American Association of Retired Persons. (1991b). *Women's financial information program.* Washington, DC: Author.

Anthony-Bergstone, C. R., Zarit, S. H., & Gatz, M. (1988). Symptoms of psychological distress among caregivers of dementia patients. *Psychology and Aging, 3,* 245-248.

Atchley, R. C. (1991). *Social forces and aging* (6th ed.). Belmont, CA: Wadsworth.

Atkinson, V. L., & Stuck, B. M. (1991). Mental health services for the rural elderly: The SAGE experience. *The Gerontologist, 31,* 548-551.

Austin, C. (1983). Case management in long-term care: Options and opportunities. *Health and Social Work, 8,* 16-30.

Austin, C. (1988, Fall). History and politics of case management. *Generations, 12,* 7-10

Balsam, A. L., & Rogers, B. L. (1991). Serving elders in greatest social and economic need: The challenge to the elderly nutrition program. *Journal of Aging and Social Policy, 3,* 41-55.

Bane, S. D. (1991). Rural minority populations. In E. P. Stanford & F. M. Torres-Gil (Eds.), Diversity: New approaches to ethnic minority aging [Special issue]. *Generations, 15*(4), 63-65.

Bane, S. D. (1992). Rural caregiving. *Rural Elderly Networker, 3*(3), 1-6.

Bartlome, J. A., Bartlome, P., & Bradham, D. D. (1992). Self-care and illness response behaviors in a frontier area. *Journal of Rural Health, 7,* 4-12.

277

Beck, S. H. (1984). Retirement preparation programs: Differentials in opportunity and use. *Journal of Gerontology, 39,* 596-602.

Beisecker, A., & Wright, L. (1991, November). *Benefits and barriers to use of ADC: Perceptions of family caregivers of individuals with Alzheimer's disease.* Paper presented at the annual meeting of the Gerontological Society of America, San Francisco.

Belden, J. N. (1992). *Housing programs and services for elders in rural America.* Kansas City, MO: National Resource Center for Rural Elderly.

Bell, W., & Revis, J. (1983). *Transportation for older Americans: Issues and options for the decade of the 1980's* (Publication No. DOT-I-83-42). Washington, DC: U.S. Department of Transportation, Office of Technology and Planning Assistance.

Berg, R. L., & Cassels, J. S. (Eds.). (1990). *The second fifty years: Promoting health and preventing disability.* Washington, DC: National Academy Press.

Bergmann, F. (1983). The future of work. *Praxis International, 3,* 308-323.

Berry, G. L., Zarit, S. H., & Rabatin, V. X. (1991). Caregiver activity on respite and nonrespite days: A comparison of two service approaches. *The Gerontologist, 31,* 830-835.

Bird, A. R. (1990). *Status of the nonmetro labor force, 1987* (Rural Development Research Report No. 79). Washington, DC: U.S. Department of Agriculture, Economic Research Service.

Blazer, D. (1989a). Affective disorders in late life. In E. Busse & D. Blazer (Eds.), *Geriatric psychiatry* (pp. 369-402). Washington, DC: American Psychiatric Press.

Blazer, D. (1989b). The epidemiology of psychiatric disorders in late life. In E. Busse & D. Blazer (Eds.), *Geriatric psychiatry* (pp. 235-262). Washington, DC: American Psychiatric Press.

Blazer, D., George, L. K., Landerman, R., Pennybaker, M., Melville, M., Woodbury, M., Monton, K. S., Jordan, K., & Locke, B. (1985). Psychiatric disorders: A rural-urban comparison. *Archives of General Psychiatry, 42,* 651-656.

Blixen, C., & Lion, J. (1991). Psychiatric visits to general hospital clinics by elderly persons and younger adults. *Hospital and Community Psychiatry, 42,* 171-175.

Bogren, S. (1991, April). Regional DHHS conferences offer solutions, barriers to coordination identified. *Community Transportation Reporter, 9,* 24.

Briley, M. E. (1989). The determinants of food choices of the elderly. *Journal of Nutrition for the Elderly, 9*(1), 39-45.

Brody, E. M., Saperstein, A. R., & Lawton, M. P. (1989). A multiservice respite program for caregivers of Alzheimer's patients. *Journal of Gerontological Social Work, 14*(1/2), 41-74.

Buckwalter, K. C. (1991). The chronically mentally ill elderly in rural environments. In E. Light & B. D. Lebowitz (Eds.), *The elderly with chronic mental illness* (pp. 216-231). New York: Springer.

Buckwalter, K. C., McLearan, H., Mitchell, S., & Andrews, P. H. (1988). Responding to mental health needs of the elderly in rural areas: A collaborative geriatric education center model. *Gerontology and Geriatrics Education, 8*(3/4), 69-80

Buckwalter, K. C., Smith, M., Zevenbergen, P., & Russell, D. (1991). Mental health services of the rural elderly outreach program. *The Gerontologist, 31,* 408-412.

Bull, C. N. (1993). *Aging in rural America.* Newbury Park, CA: Sage.

Bull, C. N., Howard, D., & Bane, S. (1991). *Challenges and solutions to the provision of programs and services to rural elders.* Kansas City, MO: National Resource Center for Rural Elderly.

Bureau of National Affairs. (1987). *Older Americans in the workforce: Challenges and solutions.* Washington, DC: Author.

Butler, R., & Newacheck, P. (1981). Health options and social factors relevant to long-term care policy. In J. Meltzer, F. Farrow, & H. Richman (Eds.), *Policy options in long term care.* Chicago: University of Chicago Press.

Bylund, R., LeRay, N., & Crawford, C. (1980). *Older American households and their housing in 1975: A metro-nonmetro comparison.* University Park: Pennsylvania State University, Agricultural Experiment Station.

Calasanti, T. M., & Hendricks, J. (1986). A sociological perspective on nutrition research among the elderly: Toward conceptual development. *The Gerontologist, 26,* 232-238.

Callahan, J. J. (1989). Play it again Sam: There is no impact. *The Gerontologist, 29,* 5-6.

Calsyn, R. (1989). Evaluation of an outreach program aimed at increasing service utilization by the rural elderly. *Journal of Gerontological Social Work, 14*(1/2), 127-135.

Capitman, J. A., Haskins, B., & Bernstein, J. (1986). Case management approaches in coordinated community-oriented long term care demonstrations. *The Gerontologist, 26*(4).

Carscaddon, D. M., George, M., & Wells, G. (1990). Rural community mental health consumer satisfaction and psychiatric symptoms. *Community Mental Health Journal, 26,* 309-318.

Center on Rural Elderly. (1991a). NCOA health promotion institute moves forward. *Bridges, 2*(2), 1.

Center on Rural Elderly. (1991b). Research identifies barriers in rural areas. *Bridges, 2*(3), 1.

Chelimsky, E. (1991). *Older Americans Act: Promising practice in information and referral services.* Washington, DC: U.S. General Accounting Office.

Clark, N. M., Becker, M. H., Janz, N. K., Lorig, K., Rakowski, W., & Anderson, L. (1991). Self management of chronic disease. *Journal of Aging and Health, 3*(1), 3-27.

Clifford, W., Heaton, T., Voss, P., & Fuguitt, G. (1985). The rural elderly in demographic perspective. In R. T. Coward & G. R. Lee (Eds.), *The elderly in rural society.* New York: Springer.

Cohen, N. L. (1992). *VENTURES: Volunteer extension trainees as unique resources for educating seniors* (Final report). Amherst: University of Massachusetts.

Colson, J. S., & Green, N. R. (1991). Effectiveness of a nutrition education program designed for sodium reduction in hypertensive versus normotensive elderly. *Journal of Nutrition for the Elderly, 11*(1/2), 31-47.

Community Nutrition Institute. (1992, July 10). Government and industry launch fruit and vegetable push; but NCI takes back seat. *Nutrition Week,* p. 1.

Cooper, J. K. (1988). A national rural geriatrics program. *Journal of Rural Health, 4,* 5-9.

Cordes, S. M. (1989). The changing rural environment and the relationship between health services and rural development. *Health Services Research Journal, 23,* 757-784.

Coward, R. T. (1979). Planning community services for the rural elderly: Implications from research. *The Gerontologist, 19,* 275-282.

Coward, R. T. (1991). Improving health care for rural elders: What do we know? What can we do? In C. N. Bull & S. D. Bane (Eds.), *The future of aging in rural America: Proceedings of a national symposium.* Kansas City, MO: National Resource Center for Rural Elderly.

Coward, R. T., Bull, C. N., Kukulka, G., & Galliher, J. (in press). *Health services for rural elders.* New York: Springer.

Coward, R. T., & Cutler, S. J. (1988). The concept of a continuum of residence: Comparing activities of daily living among the elderly. *Journal of Rural Studies, 4,* 159-168.

Coward, R. T., & Cutler S. J. (1989). Informal and formal health care systems for the rural elderly. *Health Services Research, 23,* 785-806.

Coward, R. T., Cutler, S. J., & Mullens, S. (1990). Residence differences in the composition of the helping networks of disabled elders. *Family Relationships, 39,* 44-50.

Coward, R. T., & Dwyer, J. W. (1991a). *A handbook on health programs and services for elders in rural America.* Kansas City, MO: National Resource Center for Rural Elderly.

Coward, R. T., & Dwyer, J. W. (1991b). *Health programs and services for elders in rural America: A review of life circumstances and formal services that affect the health and well-being of elders.* Kansas City, MO: National Resource Center for Rural Elderly.

Coward, R. T., & Lee, G. R. (Eds.). (1985a). *The elderly in rural society.* New York: Springer.

Coward, R. T., & Lee, G. R. (1985b). An introduction to aging in rural environments. In R. T. Coward & G. R. Lee (Eds.), *The elderly in rural society* (pp. 3-23). New York: Springer.

Coward, R. T., McLaughlin, D. K., Duncan, R. P., & Bull, C. N. (1992, September 13-15). *An overview of health and aging in rural America.* Paper presented at Health and Aging in Rural America: A National Symposium, San Diego, CA.

Coward, R. T., Miller, M., & Dwyer, J. W. (1992). The role of residence in explaining variation in reported health and dysfunction of the elderly in the United States. In National Rural Health Association (Ed.), *Study of models to meet rural health care needs through mobilization of health professions education and services resources* (pp. 529-582). Kansas City, MO: National Rural Health Association.

Cutler, S. J., & Coward, R. T. (1988). Residence differences in the health status of elders. *Journal of Rural Health, 4,* 11-26.

Cutler, S. J., & Coward, R. T. (1992). Availability of personal transportation in households of elders: Age, gender and residence differences. *The Gerontologist, 32,* 77-81.

Deimling, G. T. (1989). The respite experience. *Benjamin Rose Institute Bulletin,* third quarter, p. 1.

Deimling, G. T., & Huber, L. (1981). *The availability and participation of immediate kin in caring for the rural elderly.* Paper presented at the annual meeting of the Gerontological Society of America, Toronto.

Dorfman, L. T. (1989). Retirement preparation and retirement satisfaction in the rural elderly. *Journal of Applied Gerontology, 8,* 432-450.

Duensing, E. (1988). *America's elderly: A sourcebook.* New Brunswick, NJ: Center for Urban Policy Research.

Dunn, L. M. (1988). Respite: Preventing burnout. *Advice for Adults With Aging Parents, 2*(6), 2-4.

Dwyer, J. W. (Ed.). (1980). National conference on nutrition education: Directions for the 1980s [Special issue]. *Journal of Nutrition Education, 12*(2).

Dwyer, J. W., Lee, G. R., & Coward, R. T. (1990). The health status, health services utilization, and support networks of the rural elderly: A decade review. *Journal of Rural Health, 6,* 379-398.

Ecosometrics. (1981). *Review of reported differences between the rural and urban elderly: Status, needs, services, and service costs.* Final report to the Administration on Aging, Washington, DC.

Eggert, G. M. (1986). *Direct assessment vs. brokerage: A comparison of case management models* (Final report). Rochester, NY: Monroe County Long-Term Care, Inc.

Ehrlich, P., & White, J. (1991). TOPS: A consumer approach to Alzheimer's respite programs. *The Gerontologist, 31,* 686-691.

Erikson, L. (1991). Trends: Cultivating homegrown resources offers hope for rural America. *Inside Business, 9,* 51-53.

Evidence mounts on effectiveness of respite services. (1990, February/March). *Aging Connection,* p. 6.

FallCreek, S. (1992). *Health promotion and aging: An opportunity for advocacy.* Washington, DC: American Association of Retired Persons.

Farmers Home Administration. (1980). *Improving services for the rural elderly* (Contract No. 53-3157-9-27). Washington, DC: U.S. Department of Agriculture.

First program demonstrates success. (1992). *Respite Report, 4*(1), 4, 10.

Fitchen, J. M. (1990). Poverty as context for old age in rural America. *Journal of Rural Community Psychology, 11,* 31-49.

Fitchen, J. M. (1991). *Endangered spaces, enduring places: Change, identity, and survival in rural America.* Boulder, CO: Westview.

Flora, C. B., & Christenson, J. A. (1991). Critical times for rural America: The challenge for rural policy in the 1990s. In C. B. Flora & J. A. Christenson (Eds.), *Rural policies for the 1990s.* Boulder, CO: Westview.

Fortinsky, R. (1991). Coordinated, comprehensive community care and the Older Americans Act. In E. P. Stanford & F. M. Torres-Gil (Eds.), Diversity: New approaches to ethnic minority aging [Special issue]. *Generations, 15*(4), 39-42.

Fosmire, G. J., Manuel, P. A., & Smiciklas-Wright, H. (1984). Dietary intakes and zinc status of an elderly rural population. *Journal of Nutrition for the Elderly, 4*(1), 19-30.

Geiser, R., Hoche, L., & King, J. (1988). Respite care for mentally ill patients and their families. *Hospital and Community Psychiatry, 3,* 291-295.

Gelfand, D. E., & Olsen, J. K. (1980). *The aging network: Programs and services.* New York: Springer.

Gibbons, J., Camp, H., & Kaiser, M. (1991). Patterns of long-term care services for the rural elderly: A community approach. *Human Services in the Rural Environment, 14,* 6-11.

Ginsberg, L. H. (Ed.). (1976). *Social work in rural communities: A book of readings.* New York: Council on Social Work Education.

Glassheim, C. (n.d.). *Growing old with health and wisdom: Tailoring tips handbook.* Santa Fe: New Mexico State Agency on Aging.

Glover, E. E. (1981). Nutrition and the rural elderly. In P. K. Kim & C. P. Wilson (Eds.), *Toward mental health of the rural elderly* (pp. 97-116). Washington, DC: University Press of America.

Goldston, S. M. (1985). Adult day care homes: An alternate solution. *Perspective on Aging, 14*(6), 35.

Gonyea, J. G. (1988). Acceptance of hospital-based respite care by families and elders. *Health and Social Work, 13,* 201-208.

Goudy, W. J. (1982). Farmers, too, must plan for retirement. *Journal of Extension, 20,* 9-14.

Gunter, P. L. (1985). Four rural centers use non-traditional delivery. *Perspectives on Aging, 14*(6), 8-9, 18.

Guthrie, H. A., Black, K., & Madden, J. P. (1972). Nutritional practices of elderly citizens in rural Pennsylvania. *The Gerontologist, 27,* 330-335.

Halder, J. (1991). Bottom-up: A local approach to rural development. *Missouri Farmer, 6,* 18-19.

Hale, N. (1990). *The older worker.* San Francisco: Jossey-Bass.

Harbert, A. S., & Ginsberg, L. H. (1979). *Human services for older adults: Concepts and skills.* Belmont, CA: Wadsworth.

Harbert, W., & Wilkinson, K. (1979, January). Growing old in rural America. *Aging,* pp. 36-40.

Hargrove, D. S., & Melton, G. B. (1987). Block grants and rural mental health services. *Journal of Rural Community Psychology, 8,* 4-11.

Harrington, H., & Richardson, N. (1990). Retiree wellness plan cuts health costs. *Personnel Journal, 69*(8), 60-62.

Louis Harris & Associates, Inc. (1975). *The myth and reality of aging in America.* Washington, DC: National Council on the Aging.

Haskins, B., Capitman, J., et al. (1985). *Final report: Evaluation of coordinated community-oriented long-term care demonstration projects.* Berkeley, CA: Berkeley Planning Associates.

Hassinger, E. W. (1982). *Rural health organization: Social networks and regionalization.* Ames: Iowa State University Press.

Hausafus, C. O., Ralston, P., & DeLanoit, P. (1985). Rural older adults: Participation in and perceptions of an educational delivery system. *Educational Gerontology, 11,* 211-223.

Heffernan, W. D., & Heffernan, J. B. (1986). Impact of the farm crisis on rural families and communities. *Rural Sociologist, 6*(3), 160-170.

Heltsley, M. E. (1976). Coping: The aged in small town, U.S.A. *Journal of Home Economics, 68,* 46.

Henry, R. S. (1992, Winter). Financial lessons to be applied to new program. *Respite Report,* p. 3.

Hines, F. K., Brown, D. L., & Zimmer, J. (1975). *Social and economic characteristics of the population in metropolitan and nonmetropolitan counties* (Agricultural Economic Report No. 272). Washington, DC: U.S. Department of Agriculture, Economic Research Service.

Holahan, K. B., & Kunkel, M. E. (1986). Contribution of the Title III meals program to nutrient intake of participants. *Journal of Nutrition for the Elderly, 6*(1), 45-54.

Hollingsworth, D. S., & Hart, W. D. (1991). Effects of gender, ethnicity, and place of residence on nutrient intake among elderly residents of southwestern Louisiana. *Journal of Nutrition for the Elderly, 10*(4), 51-71.

Hoppe, R. A. (1991). *The role of the elderly's income in rural development* (Rural Development Research Report No. 80). Washington, DC: U.S. Department of Agriculture, Economic Research Service.

Hoyer, R. G. (1988, September). Urban and rural home health agencies: Some geographic differences. *Caring,* pp. 50-53.

Hughes, S. L. (1986). *Long-term care: Options in an expanding market.* Homewood, IL: Dow Jones-Irwin.

Human, J., & Watson, C. (1991). Rural mental health in America. *American Psychologist, 46*, 232-239.

Independent Transportation Management Services, Inc. (1990). *Liability insurance and the volunteer driver: An analysis of the impact of insurance availability and cost on Minnesota volunteer drivers and volunteer transportation programs.* St. Paul: Minnesota Department of Transportation.

Institute of Medicine. (1989). *Allied health services: Avoiding crises.* Washington, DC: National Academy Press.

Institute of Medicine, Division of Health Promotion and Disease Prevention. (1990). *The second 50 years: Promoting health and preventing disability.* Washington, DC: National Academy of Sciences.

Institute of Medicine, Division of Health Promotion and Disease Prevention. (1991). *Extending life, enhancing life: A national research agenda on aging.* Washington, DC: National Academy of Sciences.

Institute of Public Administration, Department of Health and Human Resources, in association with Ecosometrics, Inc. (1980). *Improving transportation services for older Americans: Executive summary.* Washington, DC: Administration on Aging.

Johnson, J. E. (1991). Health care practices of the rural aged. *Journal of Gerontological Nursing, 17*(8), 15-19.

Justice, D., & Preston, B. (1986). *State long term care programs: Summary profiles of twelve states.* Washington, DC: National Governors' Association.

Kaiser, M. A. (1991). The aged in rural America. In C. B. Flora & J. A. Christenson (Eds.), *Rural policies for the 1990s.* Boulder, CO: Westview.

Kane, R. A. (1988, Fall). Introduction. *Generations, 12*, 5-6.

Kane, R. A. (1990). What is case management anyway? In R. A. Kane, K. Urv-Wong, & C. King (Eds.), *Case management: What is it anyway?* (pp. 1-17). Minneapolis: University of Minnesota, Long-Term Care Decisions Resource Center.

Kane, R. A., Penrod, J., Davidson, G., Moscovice, I., & Rich, E. (1989). *Case management costs: Conceptual models and program descriptions* (Final report to the Health Care Financing Administration). Minneapolis: University of Minnesota, School of Public Health, Division of Health Services Research.

Kart, C. (1991). *The realities of aging.* Boston: Allyn-Bacon.

Kenney, G. M., & Dubay, L. D. (1992). Examining area variation in the use of Medicare home health services. *Medical Care, 30*(1), 43-57.

Kernaghan, S. G. (1992). *Healthy People 2000 in rural America: Hospitals and communities rally.* Chicago: American Hospital Association.

Kihl, M. (1990). *The need for transportation alternatives for the rural elderly.* Ames, IA: Midwest Transportation Center.

Kim, P. K. (1981). The low income rural elderly: Under-served victims of public inequity. In P. K. Kim & C. Wilson (Eds.), *Toward mental health of the rural elderly* (pp. 15-27). Washington, DC: University Press of America.

Kim, P. K., & Wilson, C. (Eds.). (1981). *Toward mental health of the rural elderly.* Washington, DC: University Press of America.

Kirschner Associates. (1981). *Analyses of food service delivery systems used in providing nutrition services to the elderly* (Contract No. 105-79-3012). Washington, DC: U.S. Department of Health and Human Services.

Koh, E. T., & Caples, V. (1979). Nutrient intake of low-income, black families in southwestern Mississippi. *Journal of the American Dietetic Association, 75*, 665-670.

Kohrs, M. B. (1978). Title VII nutrition program for the elderly. *Journal of the American Dietetic Association, 72,* 487-492.

Koncelik, J. A. (1982). Elements of geriatric design: The personal environment. In R. Chellis, J. Seagle, & B. Seagle (Eds.), *Congregate housing for older people.* Lexington, MA: Lexington.

Kottke, T. E. (1986). Disease and risk factor clustering in the United States: The implications for public health policy. In *Integration of risk factor interventions* (DHHS Monograph Series). Washington, DC: Government Printing Office.

Krout, J. (1983). *The organization, operation, and programming of senior centers: A national survey.* Final report to the AARP Andrus Foundation, Fredonia, NY.

Krout, J. (1984a). Knowledge of senior center activities among the elderly. *Journal of Applied Gerontology, 3,* 71-81.

Krout, J. (1984b). The organizational characteristics of senior centers in America. *Journal of Applied Gerontology, 3,* 192-205.

Krout, J. A. (1985). Senior center activities and services: Findings from a national survey. *Research on Aging, 7,* 455-471.

Krout, J. A. (1986). *The aged in rural America.* Westport, CT: Greenwood.

Krout, J. A. (1987). Rural versus urban differences in senior center activities and services. *The Gerontologist, 27,* 92-97.

Krout, J. A. (1988a). Community size differences in service awareness among elderly adults. *Journal of Gerontology, 43,* S28-S30.

Krout, J. A. (1988b). *The frequency, duration, stability, and discontinuation of senior center participation: Causes and consequences.* Final report to the AARP Andrus Foundation, Fredonia, NY.

Krout, J. A. (1988c). Rural versus urban differences in elderly parents' in-person contact with their children. *The Gerontologist, 28,* 198-203.

Krout, J. A. (1989a). *Area Agencies on Aging: Service planning and provision for the rural elderly.* Final report to the Retirement Research Foundation, Fredonia, NY.

Krout, J. A. (1989b). Rural versus urban differences in health dependence among the elderly population. *International Journal of Aging and Human Development, 28,* 141-156.

Krout, J. A. (1989c). *Senior centers in America.* Westport, CT: Greenwood.

Krout, J. A. (1990a). *Meeting the needs of rural elders: Eighty program profiles.* Kansas City, MO: National Resource Center for Rural Elderly.

Krout, J. A. (1990b). *The organization, operation, and programming of senior centers in America: A seven year follow-up.* Final report to the AARP Andrus Foundation, Fredonia, NY.

Krout, J. A. (1991a). *Case management for the rural elderly: A national analysis.* Final report to the AARP Andrus Foundation, Fredonia, NY.

Krout, J. A. (1991b, November). *Community-size differences in activities of daily living assistance among the elderly: An Upstate New York analysis.* Paper presented at the annual meeting of the Gerontological Society of America, San Francisco.

Krout, J. A. (1991c). *A guide to successful congregate programming for the elderly.* Albany: New York State Office for the Aging.

Krout, J. A. (1991d). Rural Area Agencies on Aging: An overview of activities and policy issues. *Journal of Aging Studies, 5,* 409-424.

Krout, J. A. (1992). *Rural aging community-based services.* Paper prepared for Health and Aging in Rural America: A National Symposium, San Diego, CA.

Krout, J. A., Cutler, S. J., & Coward, R. T. (1990). Correlates of senior center participation: A national analysis. *The Gerontologist, 30,* 72-79.

Krout, J. A., & Dwyer, J. W. (1991). Demographic characteristics of the rural elderly. In C. N. Bull & S. D. Bane (Eds.), *The future of aging in rural America: Proceedings of a national symposium* (pp. 5-22). Kansas City, MO: National Resource Center for Rural Elderly.

Lassey, W. R., & Lassey, M. L. (1985). The physical health status of the rural elderly. In R. T. Coward & G. R. Lee (Eds.), *The elderly in rural society.* New York: Springer.

Lawton, M. P., Brody, E. M., & Saperstein, A. R. (1989a). A controlled study of respite service for caregivers of Alzheimer's patients. *The Gerontologist, 29,* 8-16.

Lawton, M. P., Brody, E. M., & Saperstein, A. R. (1989b, November/December). Respite care for Alzheimer's families: Research findings and their relevance to providers. *American Journal of Alzheimer's Care and Related Disorders and Research,* pp. 31-38.

Lawton, M. P., & Nahemow, L. (1973). Ecology and the aging process. In C. Eisdorfer & M. P. Lawton (Eds.), *Psychology of adult development and aging.* Washington, DC: American Psychological Association.

Lazere, E., et al. (1989). *The other housing crisis: Sheltering the poor in rural America.* Washington, DC: Center on Budget and Policy Priorities, Housing Assistance Council.

Leanse, J., & Wagner, L. (1975). *Senior centers: A report of senior group programs in America.* Washington, DC: National Council on the Aging.

Learner, R. M., & Kivett, V. R. (1981). Discriminators of perceived dietary adequacy among the rural elderly. *Journal of the American Dietetic Association, 78,* 330-336.

Lebowitz, B. D., Light, E., & Baily, F. (1987). Mental health center services for the elderly: The impact of coordination with area agencies on aging. *The Gerontologist, 27,* 699-702.

Lee, C. J., Tsui, J., Glover, E., Glover, L. B., Kumelachew, M., Warren, A. P., Perry, G., Godwin, S., Hunt, S. W., McCray, M., & Stigger, F. E. (1991). Evaluation of nutrient intakes of rural elders in eleven southern states based on sociodemographic life style indicators. *Nutrition Research, 11,* 1383-1396.

Lee, E., Grant, P. R., & Gillis, D. C. (1987). Program in nutrition, consumer issues, and medication for seniors: Using a peer approach. *Canadian Home Economics Journal, 37*(2), 88-91.

Lee, J., Tamakloe, E. K. A., & Mulinazzi, T. (1981). *A public transportation needs study for the low density areas in a five-state region in the Midwest* (Final report prepared for the U.S. Department of Transportation, Urban Mass Transportation Administration, Office of Policy Research). University of Kansas, Transportation Center

Leigh, J., Richardson, N., Beck, R., Kerr, C., Harrington, H., Parcell, C., & Fries, J. (1992). Randomized controlled study of a retiree health promotion program. *Archives of Internal Medicine, 152,* 1201-1206.

Leutz, W., Greenberg, J., Abrahams, R., Prottas, J., Diamond, L., & Gruenberg, L. (1985). *Changing health care for an aging society.* Lexington, MA: Lexington.

Levinson, R. (1988). *Information and referral networks: Doorways to human services.* New York: Springer.

Levinson, R., & Haynes, K. (Eds.). (1984). *Accessing human services: International perspectives.* Beverly Hills, CA: Sage.

Lidoff, L. (1984). *Mobilizing community outreach to the high risk elderly: The "gatekeepers' approach."* Washington, DC: National Council on the Aging.

Lubben, J. E., Weiler, P. G., Chi, I., & De Jong, F. (1988). Health promotion for the rural elderly. *Journal of Rural Health, 4,* 85-96.

MaloneBeach, E. E., Zarit, S. H., & Spore, D. L. (1992). Caregivers' perceptions of case management and community-based services: Barriers to service use. *Journal of Applied Gerontology, 11,* 145-159.

Mathews, R. M., & Fawcett, S. B. (1981). *Matching clients and services: Information and referral.* Beverly Hills, CA: Sage.

May, A., Herrman, S., & Fitzgerald, J. (1976). *An evaluation of congregate meals programs and health of elders: Scott County and Fort Smith, Arkansas* (Bulletin No. 808). Fayetteville: University of Arkansas.

McCoy, J. L., & Brown, D. (1978). Health status among low-income elderly persons: Rural-urban differences. *Social Security Bulletin, 41*(6), 14-26.

McKinley, A. H., & Goodman, J. A. (1984, March). *Emerging guidelines: The Black Canyon City Project.* Intensive learning seminar presented at the annual meeting of the American Society on Aging, Denver, CO.

McKinley, A. H., & Peterson, L. (1988). *Beginning with I&R: A case management triage system* (Report from the Yavapai Regional Medical Center, Geriatrics Resource Center). Phoenix, AZ: Flinn Foundation.

Mechanic, D. (1992). General physicians' limited role in mental health care. *Hospital and Community Psychiatry, 43,* 429.

Meddin, J., & Vaux, A. (1988). Subjective well-being among the rural elderly population. *International Journal of Aging and Human Development, 27,* 193-206.

Melton, G. B., & Childs, A. W. (1983). *Rural psychology.* New York: Plenum.

Meltzer, J. W. (1982). *Respite care: An emerging family support service.* Washington, DC: Center for the Study of Social Policy.

Mental health and rural aging. (1990, March 15). *Rural Elderly Networker.*

Mercier, J. M., & Powers, E. A. (1984). The family and friends of rural aged as a natural support system. *Journal of Community Psychology, 12,* 334-346.

Mermelstein, J., & Sundet, P. A. (1986). Rural community mental health centers' response to the farm crisis. *Human Services in the Rural Environment, 10*(1), 21-26.

Miller, D. B., & Goldman, L. (1989). Perceptions of care givers about special respite services for the elderly. *The Gerontologist, 29,* 408-410.

Miller, D. B., Gulle, N., & McCue, F. (1986). The realities of respite for families, clients, and sponsors. *The Gerontologist, 26,* 467-470.

Miller, N. C., & Goodnight, J. C. (1973). *Policies and procedures for planning transit systems in small urban areas* (Transit Planning and Development, Highway Research Record, No. 449). Washington, DC: Highway Research Board.

Moak, G. S., & Fisher, W. H. (1991). Geriatric patients and services in state hospitals: Data from a national survey. *Hospital and Community Psychiatry, 42,* 273-276.

Montgomery, R. H. (1992, September 18). *Utilization of services.* Paper presented at the conference, Alzheimer's Disease: Translating Research in Policy and Practice, Portland, OR.

Montgomery, R. J. V., & Borgatta, E. M. (1989). The effects of alternative support strategies on family caregiving. *The Gerontologist, 29,* 457-464.

Multicultural respite. (1992, Fall). [Brookdale National Group Respite Program for Alzheimer's Families], *2*(2), 6.

Murray, J. D., & Keller, P. A. (1991). Psychology and rural America: Current status and future directions. *American Psychologist, 46,* 220-231.

National Association for Transportation Alternatives. (1988, March). *Equity in transportation.* Washington, DC: Author.

National Association of County Engineers. (1986). *Rural public transportation.* Washington, DC: Federal Highway Administration.

National Eldercare Institute on Transportation. (1992a). *Best practice profiles for model transportation systems serving the elderly.* Washington, DC: U.S. Department of Health and Human Services, Administration on Aging.

National Eldercare Institute on Transportation. (1992b). *Focus group report.* Washington, DC: U.S. Department of Health and Human Services, Administration on Aging.

National Information and Referral Support Center. (1991). *National standards for Older Americans Act information and referral* (Final report). Washington, DC: National Association of State Units on Aging.

National Institute on Adult Day Care. (1984). *Standards for adult day care.* Washington, DC: National Council on the Aging.

National Institute on Adult Day Care. (1990). *Standards and guidelines for adult day care.* Washington, DC: National Council on the Aging.

Native Americans use ancient tribal customs to help heal modern health problems. (1991, Fall). *Advances,* pp. 1, 12.

Nelson, G. (1980). Social services to the urban and rural aged: The experience of area agencies on aging. *The Gerontologist, 20,* 200-207.

Netting, F. E., & Kennedy, L. N. (1985). Project RENEW: Development of a volunteer respite care program. *The Gerontologist, 25,* 573-575.

North Carolina Department of Transportation, Public Transportation Division. (1979, January). *Transportation development planning for nonurbanized areas: A guide book for local governments and service providers.* Raleigh: Author.

Norton, L., & Wozny, M. C. (1984). Residential location and nutritional adequacy among elderly adults. *Journal of Gerontology, 39,* 592-595.

Office of Technology Assessment. (1990). *Health care in rural America* (Publication No. OTA-H-434). Washington, DC: Government Printing Office.

Parks, A. (1988). *Black elderly in rural America: A comprehensive study.* Bristol, IN: Wyndham Hall.

Peak, C. (1990, May). *Rural employment alternatives.* Paper presented at the Heartland Conference, Kansas City, MO.

Pennsylvania Department of Economic and Employment Development. (1989). *Single point of contact: A report for the northern tiers of counties in the state of Pennsylvania on efforts to integrate and structure public services for employment.* Harrisburg: Author.

Pepper Commission. (1990). *A call for action.* Washington, DC: Government Printing Office.

Peterson, D. (1983). *Facilitating education for older learners.* San Francisco: Jossey-Bass.

Popper, F. J. (1986). The strange case of the contemporary American frontier. *Yale Review, 76,* 101-121.

Porter, K. H. (1989). *Poverty in rural America: A national overview.* Washington, DC: Center on Budget and Policy Priorities.

Posner, B. M. (1979). *Nutrition and the elderly.* Lexington, MA: D. C. Heath.

Posner, B. M., Ohls, J. C., & Morgan, J. C. (1987). The impact of food stamps and other variables on nutrient intake in the elderly. *Journal of Nutrition for the Elderly, 6*(3), 3-16.

Preventive Services Task Force. (1989). *Guide to clinical preventive services.* Washington, DC: Government Printing Office.

Price, W. F. (1980). Developing resources of the rural elderly through education. *Educational Gerontology, 5,* 423-427.

Prosper, V. (1990a). *Housing older New Yorkers: Design features.* Albany: New York State Office for the Aging and New York State Division of Housing and Community Renewal.

Prosper, V. (1990b). *Housing older New Yorkers: Housing related preferences of older persons.* Albany: New York State Office for the Aging and New York State Division of Housing and Community Renewal.

Prosper, V. (1991). *RESTORE: An analysis and report of the RESTORE program's first two years of operation.* Albany: New York State Division of Housing and Community Renewal.

Ralston, P. (1986a, June). *Nutrition education and targeted older adult audiences: Delivery systems and methods.* Paper presented at the annual meeting of the American Home Economics Association.

Ralston, P. (1986b). Senior centers in rural communities: A qualitative study. *Journal of Applied Gerontology, 5,* 76-92.

Ralston, P., & Jones, R. (1984). The Gerontology Workshop Series: A successful effort to educate gerontology professionals in Iowa. *Gerontology and Geriatrics Education, 4,* 43-56.

Raschko, R. (1985). Systems integration at the program level: Aging and mental health. *The Gerontologist, 25,* 460-463.

Raschko, R. (1990). The gatekeeper model for the isolated, at-risk elderly. In N. L. Cohen (Ed.), *Psychiatry takes to the street.* New York: Guilford.

Rathbone-McCuan, E. (1993). Rural geriatric mental health care: A continuing service dilemma. In C. N. Bull (Ed.), *Aging in rural America.* Newbury Park, CA: Sage.

Rathbone-McCuan, E., & Coward, R. T. (1985). In A. Monk (Ed.), *Handbook of gerontological services.* New York: Van Nostrand Reinhold.

Rathbone-McCuan, E., & Bricker-Jenkins, M. (1992). Elder self-neglect: A blurred concept. In E. Rathbone-McCuan & D. Fabian (Eds.), *Self-neglecting elders: A clinical dilemma.* New York: Auburn House.

Rawson, I. G., Weinberg, E. I., Herold, J. A., & Holtz, J. (1978). Nutrition of rural elderly in southwestern Pennsylvania. *The Gerontologist, 18,* 24-29.

Reaching the caregiver. (1992, Winter). *Respite Report,* pp. 5-8.

Rhoades, E. R., Reyes, L. L., & Buzzard, G. D. (1987). The organization of health services for Indian people. *Public Health Reports, 102,* 352-355.

Riley, K., & Elder, W. (1991). Improving the financial health of rural hospitals. *Journal of Rural Health, 7,* 526-541.

Robertson, J. (1985). *Future work: Jobs, self-employment and leisure after the industrial age.* New York: Universe.

Rogers, C. R. (1991). Health and social characteristics of the nonmetro elderly. *Agriculture Outlook, 92*(4), 26-39.

Rosenheimer, L., & Francis, E. M. (1992). Feasible without subsidy? *Journal of Gerontological Nursing, 18*(4), 21-29.

Rowles, G. D. (1991). Changing health culture in rural Appalachia: Implications for serving the elderly. *Journal of Aging Studies, 5,* 375-389.

Rucker, G. (1991, April). Growth in state funding remains skewed. *Community Transportation Reporter, 9,* 4-8.

Salmon, R. (1979). The older volunteer: Personal and organizational considerations. *Journal of Gerontological Social Work, 2,* 67-77.

Sandell, S. H. (1988). Public policies and programs affecting older workers. In M. E. Borus, H. S. Parnes, S. H. Sandell, & B. Seidman (Eds.), *The older worker* (pp. 207-228). Madison, WI: Industrial Relations Research Association.

Sandell, S. H., & Baldwin, S. E. (1990). Older workers and employment shifts: Policy responses to displacement. In I. Bluestone, R. Montgomery, & J. D. Owen (Eds.), *The aging of the American workforce: Problems, programs, policies* (pp. 126-145). Detroit: Wayne State University Press.

Schauer, P. M. (1980). The typical elderly transportation provider. In Institute of Public Administration (Ed.), *Improving transportation services for older Americans.* Washington, DC: Administration on Aging.

Scheidt, R., & Norris-Baker, C. (1990). A transactional approach to environmental stress among older residents of rural communities: Introduction to a special issue. *Journal of Rural Community Psychology, 11,* 5-30.

Schneider, B. (1988, Fall). Care planning: The core of case management. *Generations, 12,* 16-18.

Schulder, D. (1985). Older Americans Act: A vast network of public, private agencies. *Perspectives on Aging, 14,* 5-7.

Schwenk, F. N. (1992). Economic status of rural older adults. *Agriculture Outlook, 92*(4), 3-14.

Secord, L. J. (1987). *Private case management for older persons and their families.* Excelsior, MN: Interstudy.

Sela, I. (1986). *A study of programs and services for the hearing impaired elderly in senior centers and clubs in the U.S.* Unpublished doctoral dissertation, Gallaudet College.

Shannon, B. M., Smiciklas-Wright, H., Davis, B., & Lewis, C. (1983). A peer educator approach to nutrition for the elderly. *The Gerontologist, 23,* 123-131.

Sharlach, A., & Frenzel, C. (1986). An evaluation of institution-based respite care. *The Gerontologist, 26,* 77-82.

Sharp, J. (1991, July). Breaking the mold: New ways to govern Texas. *Texas Performance Review, 2,* 589.

Sherman, R. H., Tirrillito, T., O'Rourke, K., & Nathanson, I. (1991, November). *New models for job training and placement of low-income older workers: Title V revisited with theory and some data.* Paper presented at the annual meeting of the Gerontological Society of America, San Francisco.

Siegel, J. (1979). Prospective trends in the size and structure of the elderly population, impact of mortality trends and some implications. In U.S. Bureau of the Census, *Current population reports* (Series P-23, No. 82). Washington, DC: Government Printing Office.

Skinner, J. (1990). Targeting benefits for the black elderly: The Older Americans Act. In Z. Harel, E. A. McKinney, & M. Williams (Eds.), *Black aged: Understanding diversity and service needs* (pp. 165-182). Newbury Park: Sage.

Smerk, G. M. (1991). Exploring topics for bus transit research. *Bus Ride, 27*(3), 56.

Smiciklas-Wright, H. (1981). Nutrition education and the elderly. *Journal of Nutrition for the Elderly, 1*(2), 3-15.

Smith, D. G., & Zuckerman, H. S. (1991). Perceptions of community leaders and the merger of rural health services. *Journal of Community Health, 16,* 83-92.

Sommers, I. (1989). Geographic location and mental health services utilization among the chronically mentally ill. *Community Mental Health Journal, 25,* 132-144.

Sorenson, A. W., & Ford, M. (1981). Diet and health for senior citizens: Workshops by the health team. *The Gerontologist, 21,* 257-262.

Sperling, D., & Goralka, R. (1988). Demand for intercity buses by the rural elderly. *Transportation Research Record, 1202,* 106-112.

Spiegel, P. B. (1990). Confidentiality endangered under some circumstances without special management. *Psychotherapy, 27,* 636-643.

Stanford, E. P. (1990). Target populations: Older Americans Act reauthorization 1991. *Minority Aging Exchange, 2*(3), 4-5, 8.

Steele, M. F., & Bryan, J. D. (1985-1986). Dietary status of elderly persons living in an urban community during winter and summer seasons. *Journal of Nutrition for the Elderly, 5,* 23-34.

Steun, C. (1985). Outreach to the elderly: Community-based services. *Journal of Gerontological Social Work, 8*(3/4), 85-96.

Stevens, D. A., Grivetti, L. E., & McDonald, R. B. (1992). Nutrient intake of urban and rural elderly receiving home delivered meals. *Journal of the American Dietetic Association, 92,* 714-718.

Stuve, P., Beeson, P. G., & Hartig, P. (1989). Trends in the rural community work force: A case study. *Hospital and Community Psychiatry, 20,* 932-936.

Taietz, P. (1970). *Community structure and aging.* Ithaca, NY: Cornell University Press.

Taietz, P., & Milton, S. (1979). Rural-urban differences in the structure of services for the elderly in Upstate New York counties. *Journal of Gerontology, 34,* 429-437.

Tardiff, T. J., Lam, T. M., & Dana, J. P. (1977). *Small city and rural transportation planning: A review* (Report No. IT-D-SR-77-2). Davis: University of California, Department of Civil Engineering.

Tausig, M. (1986). Detecting cracks in the mental health service system: Applications of network analytical techniques. *American Journal of Community Psychology, 15,* 336-351.

Teigen, T. (1991, February). Rural hospitals—forming alliances: A matter of survival. *Hospital News* [Minnesota], *2,* 20.

U.S. Bureau of the Census. (1981). *1980 Census: General social and economic characteristics* (Vol. 1). Washington, DC: Government Printing Office.

U.S. Bureau of the Census. (1983a). *1980 census of population: Characteristics of the population, United States summary* (Report No. PC 80-1-C1). Washington, DC: Government Printing Office.

U.S. Bureau of the Census. (1983b). *Census population and housing, 1980: Public use microdata samples.* Washington, DC: Government Printing Office.

U.S. Bureau of the Census. (1987). *Current population reports: Money income and poverty status of families and persons in the United States: 1986* (Series P-60, No. 157). Washington, DC: Government Printing Office.

U.S. Bureau of the Census. (1991a). *Current population reports: Poverty in the United States: 1988 and 1989* (Series P-60, No. 171). Washington, DC: Government Printing Office.

U.S. Bureau of the Census. (1991b). *Statistical abstract of the United States* (111th ed.). Washington, DC: Government Printing Office.

U.S. Department of Agriculture, Economic Research Service. (1984). New definitions for metropolitan areas (Report prepared by C. Beale). *Rural Development Perspectives, 1*, 19-20.

U.S. Department of Agriculture, Economic Research Service. (1985). *The diverse social and economic structure of nonmetropolitan America* (Rural Development Research Report No. 49). Washington, DC: Government Printing Office.

U.S. Department of Agriculture, Office of Transportation. (1989). *Reconnecting rural America: Recommendations for a national strategy.* Washington, DC: Government Printing Office.

U.S. Department of Agriculture, Transportation and Marketing Division, Agricultural Marketing Service. (1991). *Transportation in rural America: A policy backgrounder.* Washington, DC: Government Printing Office.

U.S. Department of Health and Human Services. (1988a). *Secretary's Commission on Nursing: Vol. 1. Final report.* Washington, DC: Government Printing Office.

U.S. Department of Health and Human Services. (1988b). *Secretary's Commission on Nursing: Vol. 2. Support studies and background information.* Washington, DC: Government Printing Office.

U.S. Department of Health and Human Services. (1990). *Healthy People 2000: National health promotion and disease prevention objectives* (conference ed.). Washington, DC: Government Printing Office.

U.S. Department of Health and Human Services. (1992). *The Medicare 1992 handbook.* Baltimore, MD: Health Care Financing Administration.

U.S. General Accounting Office. (1991). *Services for the elderly: Longstanding transportation problems need more federal attention* (Report No. GAO/HRD-91-117). Washington, DC: Government Printing Office.

U.S. General Accounting Office. (1982). *Comptroller general's report: Available grant funds for transportation systems in nonurbanized areas are not achieving their full impact* (Report No. GAO/CED-82-84). Washington, DC: Government Printing Office.

U.S. Senate, Committee on Agriculture and Forestry, Subcommittee on Rural Development. (1974, February). *The transportation of people in rural areas.* Washington, DC: Government Printing Office.

U.S. Senate, Special Committee on Aging. (1992). *Common beliefs about the rural elderly: Myth or fact?* Washington, DC: Government Printing Office.

Urv-Wong, K. (1990). Case management in rural areas: An overview. In R. A. Kane, K. Urv-Wong, & C. King (Eds.), *Case management: What is it anyway?* (pp. 84-104). Minneapolis: University of Minnesota, Long-Term Care Decisions Resource Center.

Urv-Wong, K., & Kane, R. A. (1989). *Case management in South Carolina: Review of practices in the South Carolina Aging Network.* Minneapolis: University of Minnesota, Long-Term Care Decisions Resource Center.

Van Hook, R. (1987). Rural health crisis for the elderly. *Rural Health Care, 9*(2), 13.

Van Werkhooven, M. V. (1991-1992). Respite care in the long-term continuum. *Journal of Long-Term Care Administration, 19,* 36-39.

Wagenfeld, M. O., Goldsmith, H. F., Stiles, D., & Manderscheid, R. W. (1988). Inpatient mental health services in metropolitan and nonmetropolitan counties. *Journal of Rural Community Psychology, 9,* 13-28.

Wallace, S. (1991). The no-care zone: Availability, accessibility, and acceptability in community-based long-term care. *The Gerontologist, 31,* 254-261.

Walzer, N., & Chicoine, D. (1989). *Rural roads and bridges: Federal and state financing.* Washington, DC: U.S. Department of Agriculture, Office of Transportation.

Watkins, D. A., & Watkins, J. M. (1985). Policy development for the elderly: Rural perspectives. In R. T. Coward & G. R. Lee (Eds.), *The elderly in rural society* (pp. 223-241). New York: Springer.

Weaver, P., Schauer, P. M., Proctor, J., & Day, S. (1991). *Supporting and encouraging general public transit ridership in Kansas.* Lawrence: University of Kansas, Transportation Center.

Webb, L. C. (Ed.). (1989). *Planning and managing adult day care.* Owings Mills, MD: National Health.

Webb, L. C., & Heide, J. (1991). *Day care programs and services for elders in rural America.* Kansas City, MO: National Resource Center for Rural Elderly.

White, M. (1987). Case management. In G. Maddox et al. (Eds.), *The encyclopedia of aging.* New York: Springer.

Williams, L., Kim, S., & McMullen, E. A. (1986). Nutrition education to facilitate dietary modification in hypertensive elderly. *Journal of Nutrition for the Elderly, 6*(2), 13-30.

Williams, M., Ebrite, F., & Redford, L. (1991). *In-home services for elders in rural America.* Kansas City, MO: National Resource Center for Rural Elderly.

Wong, H., Krondl, M., & Williams, J. I. (1982). Long-term effect of a nutrition intervention program for the elderly. *Journal of Nutrition for the Elderly, 2*(1), 31-48.

Wood, J. G., Hughes, R. G., & Estes, C. L. (1986). Community health centers and the elderly: A potential new alliance. *Journal of Community Health, 11,* 137-146.

Wright, A. D., Lund, D. A., & Caserta, M. (1990, November 13). *The use of respite services by caregivers of dementia patients: An analysis of time-use strategies.* Poster presentation at the meeting of the National Council on Family Relations, Seattle, WA.

Yearwood, A. W., & Dressel, P. L. (1983). Interracial dynamics in a southern rural senior center. *The Gerontologist, 23,* 512-517.

Youmans, E. G. (1980). The rural aged. In J. S. Quadagno (Ed.), *Aging, the individual and society: Readings in social gerontology* (pp. 213-223). New York: St. Martin's.

Young, C. L., Goughler, D. H., & Larson, P. J. (1986). Organizational volunteers for the rural frail elderly: Outreach, casefinding, and service delivery. *The Gerontologist, 26,* 342-349.

Zarit, S. H. (1992, September 17). *Relieving the burdens of caregiving: What we know from research.* Paper presented at the conference, Translating Caregiver Research into Policy and Practice, Portland, OR.

Zarit, S. H., & Teri, L. (1991). Interventions and services for family caregivers. *Annual Review of Gerontology and Geriatrics, 11,* 287-310.

Author Index

Subject Index

297

About the Authors

Robert L. Ballantyne is Director of the East Central Iowa Employment and Training Consortium in Cedar Rapids. He received his B.A. from the University of Northern Iowa (formerly Iowa State Teachers College) and his M.A. from the University of Iowa, and he served in the U.S. Peace Corps in Iran during 1969-1970. An educator by profession, he has taught at the elementary through postsecondary levels. For the past 15 years he has administered agencies and programs that provide employment and training services. He is a former Director and President of the Mid-States Employment and Training Association and a current member of the National Association of Employment and Training Administrators.

Share DeCroix Bane, M.Ed., has 20 years' experience in the field of aging. She has worked in the area of program development and design as an educator and consultant, and has developed programs in rural areas that included using senior volunteers, wellness promotion, and caregiving. She was principal trainer for the Volunteer Information Provider Program, a caregiving program designed specifically for rural communities, and coauthor of the report that came out of that program. As Director of the National Resource Center for Rural Aging at the University of Missouri—Kansas City she coordinated education, research, and technical assistance targeted to providers of services to the rural elderly. As a licensed counselor and marriage and family therapist, she has had a private practice specializing in counseling the elderly and their families.

Stockton Clark received his M.P.A. from the Maxwell School of Citizenship and Public Affairs, Syracuse University. He is currently Assistant Commissioner for Program Management for the New York State Division of Housing and Community Renewal and Vice President of the New York State Housing Trust Fund Corporation. He is Past Chair of the National Center on Rural Aging and a past board member of the National Council on Aging.

Nancy L. Cohen, Ph.D., R.D., is an Associate Professor of Nutrition at the University of Massachusetts, Amherst, and State Extension Nutrition and Food Specialist. Her research interests include studies of the effectiveness of nutrition education, assessment of dietary intake methodology, and nutrition intake of elderly blacks. She has developed many educational programs for parents, day-care providers, food handlers, adults, and elderly, including the VENTURES volunteer educator program for older adults. She is also the author of numerous home-study courses, pamphlets, newsletter articles, media programs, and fact sheets and is a frequent media spokesperson and trainer of nutrition and health professionals.

Lorraine T. Dorfman, Ph.D., is Professor in the School of Social Work at the University of Iowa, Iowa City. She has conducted research on rural retirement, academic retirement, and aging and family. She was principal investigator for the retirement substudy of the 65+ Rural Health Study, an ongoing epidemiological investigation of two rural counties in Iowa sponsored by the National Institute on Aging. Her current research interests include service utilization of retired rural elders and supports for low-income caregivers.

James M. Galliher holds a Ph.D. in sociology from the University of Arizona. Since 1990, he has been Director of the Center on Rural Elderly at the University of Missouri—Kansas City, which produces and disseminates health education resource materials for human service providers in rural and urban areas. Prior to directing the center, he was a Research Associate and Statistician with the American Nurses' Association for more than seven years. He also teaches statistics, research methods, and juvenile justice and directs graduate student research in the Department of Sociology at UMKC as an Adjunct Professor. His research interests include health and behavior, the structuring of normative phenomena and perceptions, youth and juvenile justice, and the sociology of law.

John A. Krout, Ph.D., is Professor of Health Sciences and Director, Gerontology Institute of Ithaca College. He previously was Professor of Sociology and Director of the Health Care Administration program and coordinator of the gerontology concentration at the State University of New York—College at Fredonia. He has published 30 articles in a wide range of academic journals and has made some 75 presentations at national and state conferences. He has received 10 grants to support his research program on rural aging issues, which focuses on community-based services. His books include *The Aged in Rural America* and *Senior Centers in America* as well as several bibliographies on rural aging. He has conducted national studies on senior centers, Area Agencies on Aging, and case management for the rural elderly, with the majority of his funding coming from the AARP Andrus Foundation. He currently serves as a consultant to the National Institute on Multipurpose Senior Centers and Community Focal Points and recently spent three years as a project specialist for the National Resource Center for the Rural Elderly. He has served as a member of the delegate council of the National Council on the Aging's National Center on Rural Aging. He currently serves on the boards of directors of several state and local aging organizations and on the editorial boards of *The Gerontologist* and the *Journal of Applied Gerontology,* and is a Fellow of the Gerontological Society of America.

Donna McDowell, M.S.S., is the Director of the Wisconsin Bureau of Aging, a position she has held since 1981.

Anne H. McKinley, M.S.W., has a private social work practice in Prescott, Arizona, focusing on counseling with older adults and their families and providing social work consultation in long-term care settings. She received her education at Louisiana Tech University, Tulane University, and her M.S.W. with a master's certificate in gerontology at the University of Denver. She has worked in nonprofit settings, where she has developed home- and community-based services as well as a community outreach program in a rural hospital. She has also worked as Program and Staff Specialist for the Arizona Governor's Advisory Council on Aging. Currently, she serves as adjunct faculty for the ASU School of Social Work, consults on rural issues with the University of Arizona Center on Aging, and teaches courses in social welfare policy, foundations of social work practice, and community organization for Prescott College. She has been working most recently on developing a social service and health care system on the Yavapai Prescott Indian Reservation. Her research interests include family caregiving, informal support systems, and chronic health issues in rural areas.

Robin E. Mockenhaupt, M.P.H., has a bachelor's degree in biology from the Pennsylvania State University. Her master's degree from Columbia University in public health has an emphasis in health administration and health education, and she is a certified health education specialist. She is currently Manager of the Health Advocacy Services (HAS) Section of the American Association of Retired Persons (AARP), which deals with such diverse health issues as long-term care, health promotion and wellness, advance directives and bioethics, Medicare/Medicaid and health insurance, and health consumerism. She joined the AARP staff in 1983, and was responsible for the expansion and management of the HAS volunteer program, as well as the development of many health education and advocacy programs for midlife and older persons. She also served as the Director of the National Resource Center on Health Promotion and Aging from 1988 to 1991, a grant-funded program of the Administration on Aging and AARP. She has an extensive background in health education and health promotion, and began her career by developing and implementing community health education programs in health screening, maternal and child health, and preventive medicine. She is coauthor of *Healthy Aging,* published by ABC-CLIO.

Jennifer A. Muchow, Ph.D., has been in the health promotion field for more than 13 years, most recently as the Health Promotion Program Specialist for the Center on Rural Elderly at the University of Missouri—Kansas City. She has an M.S. in biology from Bowling Green State University (Ohio) and received her doctorate in health education from the University of Toledo. From 1990 to 1993, she served as Region VII's elected representative to the Health Promotion Institute of the

National Council on the Aging. She currently serves on the national health promotion advisory council for Shepherd's Centers of America. Her professional interests include older adult health promotion, human sexuality, and women's health issues.

F. Ellen Netting, Ph.D., is Associate Professor of Social Work at Arizona State University, where she teaches in the planning, administration, and community concentration in the School of Social Work. She received her Ph.D. from the University of Chicago in 1982, her M.S.W. from the University of Tennessee in 1975, and her B.A. from Duke University in 1975. She is a member of the Aging and Adult Development Advisory Council and has taught aging policy in the aging certificate program. Her practice experience includes directing a rural office on aging and senior center, designing training and continuing education for a 16-county Area Agency on Aging network, and directing a foster grandparent program. Her current research interests focus on health, housing, and human service delivery issues for the elderly.

Ollie Owen, a widow living in Syracuse, New York, is the mother of four children and eleven grandchildren and currently retired, but still very active in the community. She organized and coordinated the first older adult county outreach program in New York State in 1972 and worked for the Metropolitan Commission on Aging (City of Syracuse and Onondaga County in New York State) for 13 years as Senior Clubs and Centers Coordinator. She served the New York State Conference on Aging in the positions of Secretary, Vice President, and President (two separate terms) and received the Henrietta Rabe Award for dedicated service to senior centers in New York State. In addition, she was an elected seven-year delegate representing New York State to the National Institute of Senior Centers, and in that capacity served on the Policy Committee of the National Council of Aging. She received honorable mention for the National Institute of Senior Centers Founders Award in 1992. From 1986 to 1990 she was a Research Associate with the Syracuse University Adult Education Department's Kellogg Project, working with computers and the elderly locally and through Seniornet, an international electronic communication network for older adults.

Vera Prosper, C.S.W., is the Housing Policy and Program Analyst for the New York State Office for the Aging. She has an M.S.W. from the State University of New York at Albany and a B.S. degree in business administration from the Pennsylvania State University. She has conducted research and published on a variety of senior housing topics, and has worked as a volunteer for numerous community housing and service organizations and agencies.

Penny A. Ralston, Ph.D., is currently Dean, College of Human Sciences, Florida State University. A native of Indiana, she received a B.S. degree from Ball State University and the M.Ed. and Ph.D. degrees from the University of Illinois. Her previous positions include Professor in the Department of Home Economics Education at Iowa State University and Professor and Chair of the Department of Consumer Studies at the University of Massachusetts. Her research interests have included community-based organizations for the elderly, health promotion and nutrition, and minority elderly issues. The bulk of her research has focused on the development and use of senior centers by the elderly. Her most recent research (with Nancy Cohen), which was funded by the AARP Andrus Foundation, concerned factors influencing dietary quality of elderly blacks. Her work has been published in the *Journal of Gerontology, The Gerontologist,* and *Journal of Applied Gerontology,* among others. She is on the editorial board of the *Journal of Nutrition for the Elderly.* She is a Fellow in the Gerontological Society of America and is currently on the board of directors of the American Home Economics Association.

Eloise Rathbone-McCuan, Ph.D., is the Associate Chief, Social Work Service, at the Colmery-O'Neil Veterans Administration Medical Center in Topeka, Kansas. She does applied geriatric mental health research and program planning in the care of the chronic mentally ill elderly in community and institutional settings. As the author of several books and numerous scientific articles on aging she has made contributions that are important to both clinical and program development. She is a Fellow in the Gerontological Society of America.

Linda J. Redford, Ph.D., R.N., is a Research Associate with the Center on Aging at the University of Kansas Medical Center, an Adjunct Professor with the School of Nursing there, and a National Kellogg Fellow. She is also coprincipal investigator of an NIA-funded study of long-term care and caregiving among the Navajo. She has worked as a community health nurse and has taught in nurse practitioner- and master's-level gerontological clinical nurse specialist programs. She has served as Associate Director of the Long-Term Care Gerontology Center at the University of Kansas Medical Center and as Project Director of the NAMFE program, a federal grant project aimed at educating nurses in assessment and care management of the frail elderly. She speaks frequently at national meetings on long-term care issues relating to rural and urban elderly. She is active in a number of aging organizations and has served on the boards of the Mid-America Congress on aging and the National Council on the Aging. She is Past Chair of the National Institute on Community-Based Long-Term Care, a constituent unit of the National Council on the Aging.

Peter M. Schauer, M.A., M.R.P., is a management consultant and transportation futurist who has provided planning, evaluation, feasibility, training, and advisory services to clients in 47 states. For 6 years he was general manager of a 100-plus vehicle system that received the UMTA (FTA) Administrator's Award for Excellence. For the past 14 years he has successfully completed projects for federal agencies, state and local governments, and private nonprofit and for-profit clients. He holds a B.S. degree from the University of Missouri and M.A. and M.R.P. (master of regional planning) degrees from the Pennsylvania State University. He is a member of the Transportation Research Board.

Vicki L. Schmall, Ph.D., has worked since 1978 as the Gerontology Specialist/Professor with Oregon State University Extension Service. She is also currently coordinating the Senior Series Project in the 17 western states/territories for the Western Rural Development Center at Oregon State University. Prior to her current position, she was the Director of the University Gerontology Program. She develops educational programs and materials on various aspects of aging for families faced with decisions about older relatives, for practitioners who work with the elderly, and for senior adults. The author of numerous publications, she has also developed four educational games on aging, five training manuals for providers, and a series of eight multimedia educational programs that have been distributed throughout the United States and Canada. She serves on the Board of Directors for the Alzheimer's Association in Portland and the Benedictine Nursing Center, Mt. Angel, Oregon. She is a Trainer for the American College of Health Care Administrators and for the American Association of Homes for the Aging Retirement Housing Managers Certification Program.

Alison B. Severns, R.N., M.S., received both her bachelor's degree and her master's degree in nursing from the University of Oklahoma, Oklahoma City, and was selected in 1991 as a Kellogg National Fellow. She served as coordinator for an early childhood intervention grant awarded by the Oklahoma Regents for Higher Education. She was responsible for providing educational services to people involved in the care of special needs children. Since her career began in 1981, she has filled many nursing roles, including that of Public Health Nurse for the Oklahoma City-County Health Department. Additionally, she has taught at the University of Oklahoma College of Nursing. She helped develop and implement Concerned Citizens for a Canadian County Health Department, a voter awareness campaign that helped to pass the millage that funded the new health department. Her numerous professional memberships include the American and Oklahoma Nurses' Association, the Oklahoma Association of Community and Junior Colleges, and the Higher Education Association of Central Oklahoma.

Ene Kristi Urv-Wong, M.H.A., is a long-term care consultant practicing in the U.S. Northwest. She holds a master's degree in hospital and health care administration from the University of Minnesota. Her primary research interests include long-term care strategic planning, case management program development, and ethics. Her experience includes coordinating the National Long-Term Care DECISIONS Resource Center at the University of Minnesota; directing education and training at the Hillhaven Foundation; health care administration positions in Seattle, Philadelphia, and Minneapolis; and work as a legislative researcher. Her publications include chapters in *Everyday Ethics: Resolving Dilemmas in Nursing Home Life* and *Values and Ethics for a Caring Staff in Nursing Homes,* a training curriculum for nurse's aides.

Patricia Weaver is Associate Research Scientist at the University of Kansas Transportation Center in Lawrence, Kansas, where she has worked since 1982. Her responsibilities at the University of Kansas include research, training, and technical assistance to rural and specialized transportation providers. Her research and training interests include transportation planning, transportation options for the elderly and disabled, local and statewide transportation coordination and funding, and microcomputer applications for transit management. She has managed a number of projects funded by the Federal Transit Administration, states, and local governments. She is program manager for the

Kansas Rural Transit Assistance Program, funded by the Federal Transit Administration; she is also program manager for the Kansas Technology Transfer Program for Rural Transportation, funded by the Federal Highway Administration. Prior to taking her current position, she worked for two years as a Technical Assistance Specialist for the Regional Education and Training Project (funded by the U.S. Administration on Aging) at the University of Kansas, providing training and technical assistance to aging network personnel in a four-state area.

Linda Cook Webb, M.S.G., has worked in adult day care for 13 years and in long-term care for 20 years. She consults with adult day care centers in development, financing, marketing, facilities planning, and programming. She also offers training to adult day care associations. She is coauthor of *Planning and Managing Adult Day Care: Pathways to Success* and *Day Care Programs and Services for Elders in Rural America*. She was twice elected Region VII representative to the Steering Committee of the National Institute on Adult Daycare (NIAD). She served as Chair of NIAD's Conference and Training Committee and sat on a board committee of the National Council on the Aging. She helped to start adult day care associations in Kansas and Missouri and served on the state of Missouri's task force to write adult day care certification and licensing standards. She earned the master of science in gerontology at the University of Southern California (Andrus Gerontology Center).

Margaret M. Williams, R.N., served as the Director of Madison County Office for the Aging (a nonprofit agency) from its inception in 1977 until February 1989. During that time, more than 20 specialized programs that serve older people were designed, funded, and implemented. Several of these programs have been used as models in New York State and nationally. From 1989 to 1990, she served as the Vice President/Administrator of Bethany Retirement Home and Community Services in Horseheads, New York. She administered a licensed adult care facility, a licensed child day-care program, a nursery school, and the Madison County Office for the Aging. She also conducted forums and workshops for the public and for professionals. In January 1991 she became the first Executive Director of the New York State Association of Area Agencies on Aging, representing 59 AAAs. She currently serves as the Executive Director of the Alzheimer's Association of Central New York.